Thirty-Seven Years Ago
My Doctor Told Me
I Had Three Years
to Live

Thirty-Seven Years Ago My Doctor Told Me I Had Three Years to Live

Reginald L. Jensen

iUniverse, Inc.

New York   Bloomington

Thirty-Seven Years Ago My Doctor Told Me I Had Three Years to Live

iUniverse books may be ordered through booksellers or by contacting:

iUniverse
1663 Liberty Drive
Bloomington, IN 47403
www.iuniverse.com
1-800-Authors (1-800-288-4677)

ISBN-13: 978-0-595-35781-9 (pbk)
ISBN-13: 978-0-595-80400-9 (cloth)
ISBN-13: 978-0-595-80250-0 (ebk)
ISBN-10: 0-595-35781-4 (pbk)
ISBN-10: 0-595-80400-4 (cloth)
ISBN-10: 0-595-80250-8 (ebk)

Printed in the United States of America

I wish to express my thanks to my wife, Dorothy, for her patience during my lifetime and for her editorial assistance in the preparation of this book.

My three daughters (Wendy Sabin, Cynthia Campbell, and Leslie Morrison) and four grandchildren (Robert Sabin, Rachel Sabin, Angela Morrison, and Anastasia Morrison) are terrific people. It's my reward and pleasure to see them all grow up.

I'd also like to thank iUniverse for its help in publishing this book

Contents

PREFACE 2010

My book *Thirty-Seven Years Ago My Doctor Told Me I Had Three Years To Live*, published in 2005, isn't full of excitement and thrills. Thankfully, it's brief. The story it tells is that a person must do more than begin an exercise regimen, that person must maintain the regimen for life. I've never stopped exercising and that's the thrust of the book.

Why should a person maintain an exercise routine if that person looks good, feels good, and has no apparent health problem? Because those looks and feelings disappear quickly. Exercising is a habit and habits need to be maintained. Not exercising is also a habit, so they need to be exchanged. What's the reward? Eventually, we all get sick, develop some disease, have a chronic medical problem, such as cancer, heart disease, Alzheimer's, diabetes, depression, and many contract a venereal disease. When a person treats the body as important many of these problems never occur.

In the article "A Thought for Tax Day: The Real Crisis Is Yet To Come,"[1] an interview with Kent Smetters, formerly deputy assistant Treasury secretary and economist for the Congressional Budget Office, explains that the current value of all property in the United States is about $55 trillion. The present value of our nation's medical expenses is approximately $80 trillion. Add to those social security obligations of about $12 trillion and our national debt of about $11 trillion. Those expenses exclude running the government, infrastructure maintenance and the rest. The nation's debt exceeds its assets by a factor of two.

The Cooper Clinic study "Effects of Cardiorespiratory Fitness on Healthcare Utilization"[2] demonstrates we can reduce medical care costs

---

1   http://www.knowledge@wharton.mht April 15, 2009
2   Mitchell, Tedd L. et. al., The Cooper Clinic, Dallas, TX. "Medicine and Science in Sports & Exercise," Copyright © 2004 by the American College of Sports Medicine.

by more than 50% if we engage in moderate exercise like walking for 20 to 30 minutes a day five days a week. That would cut the nation's medical debt in half to about $40 trillion. If we will eat right that will cut the medical debt in half again, to about $20 trillion.[3] Exercising dramatically reduces diabetes and eliminates it in many cases. The BBC News reported that exercise cuts Alzheimer's risk by 37%.[4] (Take your parents for a daily walk.) Physical activity doubles the survival rate from breast cancer.[5] Exercising prior to contracting breast cancer reduces the contracting rate by 50%. Exercising eliminates depression.[6]

According to the Centers for Disease Control and Prevention about 80 million people in the United States had venereal disease in 2005.[7] There were about 19 million new cases in 2005. The direct estimated costs associated with sexually transmitted diseases are about $14.1 billion yearly. Most of the new cases are between the ages of 15 to 24. If these young people were aware of their bodies they would protect themselves and venereal disease would drop dramatically. They would be inclined to find and stay with one partner.

Dr. Kenneth Cooper was the author of the book Aerobics (Bantom, 1968). He owns and operates the Cooper Aerobics Center in Dallas, Texas. In his biography he said "It's easier to maintain good health through proper exercise, diet, and emotional balance than to regain it once it is lost." This is proven by scientific research. The Institute's landmark eight year study of 13,000 patients showed that individuals with sedentary lifestyle are four times as likely to die from cardiovascular disease as those who exercise regularly.[8]

The new national health care plan signed by President Obama in 2010 neither reduces demand nor increases supply for medical care. In fact,

---

3   White, Russell D., with Carl Sherman. "Exercise in Diabetes Management." The Physician and Sportsmedicine. Vol. 4 – No. 27 – April 1999.

4   http://newsvote.bbc.co.uk/mpapps/pagetools/print/news.bbc.co.uk/1/hi/health/4616502.stm. 6/10/2007.

5   Holmes, Michelle D., et. al. "Nurses Health Study" Framingham, MA. Journal of the American Medical Association, Vol. 293 No. 20, May 25, 2005.

6   International Journal of Sports Medicine. No. 3, Volume 22, April 2001, Page 165-244.

7   CDC Std Surveillance 2005. http://www/cdc.gov/std/stats/trends2005.htm

8   http://www.cooperaerobics.com/corporate/biokencooper.aspx.

it increases demand and supply remains level. If the health care plan were to be modified so that we had two options, A or B, we could cut health care costs dramatically and improve health dramatically. We could assign whatever amount of money is now being spent on health care and pay 100% of all costs for the A members. The A members must engage in moderate exercise five days a week, such as a brisk 20 or 30 minute walk. The A group would include those who can't exercise for any reason. The B group would consist of those who refuse to exercise on a regular basis. The B group would receive the same medical cost benefits that the A group receives, but would be required to pay out-of-pocket the additional costs of the B group. A person could move from the B group to the A group simply by starting an exercise routine. Those who cheat would stay in the B group for at least a year. Currently, the A group's monthly cost per person would be between $100 and $200. The B group's costs per person would be about $1,000. No one would be required to join either group, but the A group would fill up since the current monies now being spent would pay their entire cost. Those people with chronic illnesses would move to the A group to reduce their medical costs. They would also contribute to their own well being and reduce the need for medical care.

On April 2, 2010, President Obama said that national bankruptcy is the future if our health care problem isn't solved. Reducing demand is the only viable solution.

When you read my book you'll find that I not only began exercising, but I continued. In 2010 my years alive since 1967 when I began exercising are forty-two. One other thought, an employee with the United States Department of Labor and another with the California Department of Labor advised me that an employer can require an employee to take a daily walk on company time. It's worth it to the employer because productivity will increase by 25% to 50%. I make this statement from my own personal experience.

Reginald L. Jensen

FOREWORD

Every once in a while someone says something or does something that has a dramatic effect on our lives. Quite often it doesn't seem important at the time, but later on we recall what was said or what happened, review the effects, and feel grateful for the event. Sometimes it does seem important at the time. Sometimes we say to ourselves, "I'm not going down that road," or "I am going down that road." We make permanent changes.

One purpose of this book is to get you to exercise. Terrible, you say? You don't want to go out and get all sweaty for nothing when you're already healthy. *All a healthy person needs to do to maintain excellent health is to walk for twenty minutes (a mile is about twenty-five to thirty minutes) five days a week. That's all. So, if you're healthy, why should you walk for twenty minutes a day?* Medical experts Tedd L. Mitchell, Larry W. Gibbons, Susan M. Devers, and Conrad P. Earnest at the Cooper Clinic in Dallas, Texas,[1] conducted a nineteen-year test of healthy males, ages twenty to seventy-nine, who exercised regularly versus those who did not exercise regularly and found the healthcare costs for those who exercised were reduced by 53%. *What? Healthy people reduce their medical expenses 53% over a nineteen-year period? What does that mean?* It simply means that some people who could have had a heart attack, didn't. People who could have developed cancer, didn't. People who could have developed diabetes, didn't. People who could have had a stroke, didn't. *Think of the lives that could have been ruined, but weren't ruined, by health problems.* Many of those people in the above study lived a healthy, rewarding life when they could have suffered unnecessary illnesses. It isn't hard to walk for twenty minutes and the benefits are so great, why not do it? Take care of your

---

1.   Mitchell, T.L., L. W. Gibbons, S. M., Devers, and C.P. Earnest, <u>Effects of Cardio-respiratory Fitness on Healthcare Utilization</u>. Copyright © 2004 by the American College of Sports Medicine; 2004, Dallas, TX, 2088-2092.

own body. You'll just plain feel a whole lot better. Don't rely on the help of a doctor or a pill until you've done everything you can do for yourself. As a bonus, think of the money you and your family will save on medical expenses.

A recently published study in the *Journal of the American Medical Association*[2] showed that breast cancer patients who walk or do other moderate exercises for three to five hours a week are about 50 percent less likely to die from the disease than sedentary women. This is the result for women after they develop breast cancer. Think of all of the lives that are being and can be saved. According to the San Jose Mercury News,[3] "Previous research has shown regular exercise reduces the chances of developing many diseases, among them heart disease and various forms of cancer, including breast cancer." Studies show how people reduce or eliminate the use of medication for diabetes by walking. Studies also show that exercise reduces feelings of depression.[4]

Another purpose of this book is to demonstrate how to avoid premature death from heart attacks. Today, according to the American Heart Association,[5] there are about sixty-five million people in the United States who have heart disease. How can heart disease be detected? By a simple blood pressure test. If a person has high blood pressure, that person probably has heart disease. Heart disease can be hereditary, a result of too much body fat, smoking, and other causes. It can begin at any age. Heart disease can be arrested. I'm just one person, not an amalgamation of a massive study, but I'm convinced many people can achieve the same results I've achieved. Walking wouldn't be enough for me. However, it isn't necessary for most people to exercise as strenuously as I do. I had to strengthen my heart muscle and lungs. As far as I am concerned, I had no choice. I had to jog. Anyone who has high blood pressure or cancer or some other debilitating

---

2.   Holmes, Michelle, D. MD, et. al., "Physical Activity and Survival After Breast Cancer." *JAMA*. Vol. 293, No. 20, May 25, 2479-2486.

3.   Stein, R., Reporter, The Washington Post, "Exercise shown to increase survival from breast cancer." The San Jose Mercury News, May 25, 2005, 7A,

4.   Blackman, H., J. Kaprio, U. Kujala, and S. Sarna. International Journal of Sports Medicine; April 2001, 219.

5.   http://www.americanheart.org/presenter.jhtml?identifier=4621. 5 July 2005.

illness should give serious thought to following my routine. But as you should do with any new exercise routine or dramatic change in activity, *check with your doctor to determine the most appropriate forms of activity for you, especially if you're ill.* Your doctor should help you with your schedule and provide needed medication.

This book chronicles what I went through when I arrested my heart disease. It wasn't easy; it was hard on my body. The easiest part was establishing the discipline necessary to accomplish the deed. Exercising, eating right, and getting the proper amount of rest became a lifestyle, not a temporary "test" to see if it works. I understood that I had two alternatives, shaping up or selecting my grave site. I chose shaping up. Many people who are told they have heart disease pick out their grave site because they believe there is no alternative, or that the alternative of a healthy lifestyle is too hard.

President John F. Kennedy advised Americans to get healthy. Physicians give the same advice. Sometimes a child watches what happens to a parent and decides that being healthy is important. Others are quick learners. When they're told that they must exercise, eat right, and get plenty of rest, they accept the advice as true and follow the course. Some people, like me, need shock treatment.

What about eating right? How does a person control weight? *Since a person's weight is controlled by the amount of food a person eats, you need to know how much you eat now before you can begin eating less.* I discuss this in Part IV. Weight control is very easy.

It seems to me that exercising, eating right, and getting the proper amount of rest are requirements of living, not options. Slipshod habits in any of these areas can mean a person has lost control over his or her own body. You are the only person who can control your body. Your body is your private temple. It doesn't do your body any good if your spouse, child, or friend exercises. It really isn't hard to manage your body successfully over the long term. You'll be amazed at how rewarding it is to have a healthy body.

Did you take physical education in high school? Were you actually taught the lifelong process of creating and maintaining a healthy body?

For me, physical education was playing sports or tossing a ball around or just sitting and watching someone else play a game. There are many physical education classes, but few teachers, if any, who've learned the process and are currently teaching what they have learned to help others develop a healthy lifestyle. Physical Education is the process of learning how to take care of your body in a systematic, rewarding manner. We learn reading, writing, and arithmetic in school but not physical education. Physical education should be properly taught.

Finally, put this book on your shelf where you can read the title as a reminder that you need to exercise on a regular basis for the rest of your life.

Reginald L. Jensen

Part I
The Thirty-Seven Years

Thirty-seven years ago, in August 1967 in Salem, Oregon, when I was thirty-six years old, I went to see my doctor, Harmon T. Harvey, who was a close personal friend. I met with him in his office on a day when I felt completely exhausted. I had no energy and even had difficulty driving to his office to meet with him. He took my blood pressure and recorded it about 260/140. He had me lie down on a couch in his office and asked me to rest. I slept for several hours. When I woke up, Dr. Harvey gave me some medication, but said there was very little he could do beyond the medication. He told me that I had only three years to live. At that time, I weighed 225 pounds and was 6 feet tall. I was married. My wife and I had three beautiful daughters, and I was an officer in a small, young life insurance company.

Salem is the capital of Oregon. My wife and I moved to Salem during the middle of the winter from the desert of Salt Lake City, Utah, in 1959. When we first entered Salem in January, we thought we'd just entered paradise. Rhododendrons were in bloom. Flowers and greenery were sprouting everywhere. Interstate 5 was landscaped with greenery and there were blossoms all the way from Portland to Salem. In the spring, the birds would eat the berries on the plants, get drunk, and fall all over the freeway. A few lost their lives. The Willamette River (pronounced will-am'-it) runs from southern Oregon north through Salem, to Portland and into the Columbia River. The natives knew what a treasure they owned. They were convinced the Willamette Valley belonged only to them. One of our neighbors volunteered the information that we shouldn't talk to him and other Oregonians until we'd lived in the state for at least ten years. Salem is an old town with beautiful small hills and, at that time, a brand new state capital. As the state capital, Salem was filled with politicians. And in the middle of all these politicians stood one honest and honorable attorney, Tom Churchill. Tom and his wife, Marian, became lifelong friends. We loved the city then and we still do. We met some of the finest people in Salem.

My mother and father were born in Norway, but did not meet until they were in the United States. My father, Harold A. Jensen Sr., was born in Bergen and was shipped to Ellis Island alone at age thirteen in 1917. No one met him in the United States and after nearly one month on Ellis Island he was put on a train to central Canada to meet his brother. He worked with his brother on a farm for several months. The farmer couldn't afford to pay my father so he and his brother parted company. When my father was about age fifteen, he walked from Canada to Lovell, Wyoming, to meet a sister. When he arrived in Lovell, his clothes were in shreds and he hadn't seen bath water in a long time. Later, he went to Goshen, Idaho and then he moved to Salt Lake City, Utah.

My mother, Ragnhild Laura Jensen (I was named after my mother), was born in Vardo (in the Arctic Circle), later moved to Bergen, and, when she was eleven years old, she shipped from Oslo to Ellis Island with her twelve-year-old sister, Ingrid (Olsen), in 1917. My mother traveled to Shelley, Idaho. She and my father eventually met in Goshen, Idaho. My parents married in 1923 and settled in Salt Lake City. My father held several different common laborer jobs before training himself to be a house painter and paperhanger. My parents gave birth to eleven children, seven boys and four girls. In order of birth they are: Harold A. Jr. (1924), Hyrum Conrad (1926), Thelma Ruth (1928), me (November 9, 1930), Leo Walter and Louis Vern (twins; 1933), David (1935), Bertha Rose (1936), Synnove Jewel (1940), and Junius and Constance (twins; 1945).

My father's death was the result of a heart attack on May 10, 1951, at age forty-seven. He had several heart attacks before the fatal event. My brothers, Harold, Conrad (now retired Lt. Col.), Leo, and Louis, have had heart problems. Heart disease and cancer seem to be genetic in our family, at least on the male side.

I met my wife, Dorothy Helen Matthes, in 1953 in the shoe department at Sears Roebuck in Salt Lake City, Utah, during the Christmas season. I was a shoe salesman and Dorothy worked part time selling house slippers. We married on Friday, May 13, 1955. We are still married and our children are Wendy Ruth (Sabin), August 28, 1951; Cynthia Lee (Campbell), September 18, 1956; and Leslie Gail (Morrison), April 28, 1959. Our four grandchildren are Robert Edward Sabin, Rachel Marie Sabin, Angela Brooke Morrison, and Anastasia Marie Morrison.

So, I was supposed to be dead by age thirty-nine. What could I do under these conditions? What are the options? Most people don't pay any attention to their bodies, just like I wasn't; they seem to believe it is what they were born with and if it conks out on them, well, that's the way it is. Some people search for a pill as the solution. Others might exercise for a short period of time hoping that will solve any medical problem. I immediately applied for a $1 million life insurance policy. My company was required to reinsure the bulk of the coverage with a larger and much older company. The reinsurance company required a medical examination from a different doctor. After reviewing my physical condition, the reinsurance company informed my company they would not issue any insurance coverage under any conditions. Life insurance protection for the benefit of my family was out of the question. My final decision was to find a way to stay alive, to place my personal health above my desire to make money.

I had reached the conclusion at that time of my life that my mind is somehow different from my brain and my body. My mind seems to operate independently from my body. For example, my body can complain of any injustice imposed upon it, but my mind can tell my body that it's complaints will go unheeded. Neither my body, nor its complaints to my brain were going to be in charge. My mind had to take over. The instructions given by my mind to my brain would have to counter the habits developed by my body.

I was a heavy smoker and a heavy drinker at that time. Smoking and drinking to excess can reduce a person's life span by seven to fifteen years. So that would have put my life expectancy to be somewhere between age sixty and sixty-five. My problem was heart disease.

My lifestyle was obviously wrong. Habits developed over thirty-six years are very hard to change. Smoking is a habit, so is drinking alcohol. Working the long hours and the work methods I employed were also habits. Eating rich and fatty foods had become a habit. I loved bacon, pork rinds, beef jerky, anything fatty. I also enjoyed staying up drinking alcohol and smoking cigarettes until the wee hours of the morning. Changes were now in order.

I was active in sports in high school and knew that exercise would improve anyone's health. I played football and basketball and a little bit of track. I could run sprints and do the long jump, but I was terrible at hurdles and high jumping. I became a participant in sports because I liked the competition. I had very little coaching. High school coaches in small towns like St. Anthony, Idaho, (where I attended high school for a couple of years) have too many duties to be able to give individual attention to the players. I remembered going with our track team to a local meet and the coach asked me to enter the mile race as a filler in an open spot. I agreed, even though I'd never run a mile race. At the sound of the gun, I ran as fast as I could and led the pack by a good distance after seven-eighths of a mile. But then I had to stop, I couldn't finish the race. Later in the year I ran a cross country race and found that speed and stamina must be combined. This was my total experience with running, but I learned that a person had to be in good shape to be a runner.

I knew that I must exercise. If my exercise required a partner, then the absence of my partner would be an excellent reason for me to skip the exercise. If I was going to take control of my body, it was necessary to engage in exercises that required no other person as part of the routine. Some of these exercises are swimming, bicycling, and jogging. Jogging seemed to me to be the best because I could jog at any time and at any location.

In the middle of September 1967, I decided to start jogging so that I could monitor my body and establish specific controls over what I intended to accomplish. I joined the YMCA in Salem. The Y had a small jogging track. The track measured about 33 to 36 laps to the mile. I say "about" because no one seemed to know for sure. I bought a pair of tennis shoes, shorts, and a T-shirt, and got on the track. I jogged very slowly around the track and made three laps. I was exhausted and had to stop and sit for a few minutes to catch my breath. I sat down on the edge of the track trying to breathe and wondering *"Oh my, am I going to survive."* That little bit of jogging made me so tired and breathless that my body ached. Eventually, I got back up and jogged a couple of laps and walked several laps. Then I jogged a lap and then walked for several more laps. After about ten minutes I stopped, showered, and went home. When I arrived home I just sat in my chair for a long time trying to recoup my energy. It had been many years since I'd felt so beat up. I smoked a couple of cigarettes, had a couple of drinks, and finally ate dinner. I went to bed early that night.

A couple of days later I went back to the jogging track at the Y and went through the same horrible, exhausting experience. This was a moment of truth for me. I knew the alternative was death, so I made a firm commitment to jog for no less than five years. That would get me past my three year life expectancy. I could see there was going to be a lot of pain and agony for me to go through. I could see no alternative in spite of the terrible strain on my body. My decision was irreversible. For me, a disciplined commitment to a course of action means the action will be completed. There might be other people who've started from a more disadvantaged position than I, but I've never met any except my brother Harold. All other joggers I've met could cover more distance with less pain when they began jogging than I could when I started. I had to steel my nerves every time I went to the Y to try jogging once more. I'd get on the track and force myself to jog. I gradually increased the laps so that I could jog four, five, then six laps without stopping.

When I first began I would jog late in the day before dinnertime. Each day after jogging, I'd come home, sit in my chair to read the paper, smoke a cigarette, and have a drink. After about three months my eyes responded differently. As I sat in my chair I would see thousands of little sparkles about three feet in front of my eyes. It was as if someone lighted a fourth of July sparkler and the remnants sprang out in front of me. I had been consulting a psychiatrist, Dr. Ian MacLaughlin, in Portland, Oregon, and told him about the sparklers. Dr. MacLaughlin said he believed the nicotine from the cigarettes was settling in the veins in my feet and legs and my jogging was breaking the nicotine loose. He said that if he was right, I would eventually lose my feet because gangrene would set in. That was the end of my smoking. I threw away the balance of my pack of cigarettes when I left his office and have never smoked since.

About three months after I quit smoking I decided to cut back on the alcohol. I decided to drink only on Friday and Saturday nights. I'd drink all the alcohol I could consume on those nights and none during the rest of the week. *It soon became obvious to me that I felt good on the week days and terrible on the weekends.* So I reduced the drinking to Saturday nights only. *After another five or six Saturdays it was so obvious how much better I felt without alcohol in my system that I was convinced to put alcohol out into the same pasture with nicotine.* I've never consumed alcohol since.

About nine months after I started jogging, I read an article in a Salem newspaper about *Aerobics* (later retitled *The Aerobics Way*), a book by Dr. Kenneth Cooper, in which various methods of maintaining and measuring physical fitness are analyzed. I bought the book and highly recommend it. It has more detail than anyone will ever need. One of Dr. Cooper's guidelines for jogging at my age was to cover two miles in sixteen minutes. That became my first goal.

I changed my schedule to jogging just before lunch. I would jog, eat lunch, and go back to work. If I had an appointment to meet a person right after lunch, the other person would usually comment on my red face, or I'd tell the person that I had been jogging just a short time before we met. They always answered, "I can see that." For quite a few months my face would show the redness for an hour or so after my exercise.

Over the weeks and months my jogging got a little bit easier each time. I was making progress. My jogging routine was three times a week, covering two miles in any fashion. I thought that if I needed to lie down and roll part of the distance, then I'd do it. After about six months I could jog a mile very slowly without stopping. Then I'd walk for awhile and jog several more times until I finished the two miles. After a year my time for two miles was about thirty minutes, and it was still an exhausting ordeal. I told

Dr. MacLaughlin how exhausted I was after jogging. He said that if I slowed down it should be a little easier. I told him that I did slow down, but I was still just as exhausted. Going slower or faster seemed to make no difference. He said he didn't understand why. Still, I kept at it and it was more than a year before I could jog two miles without stopping. One day I was walking along a park just south of downtown Salem and two joggers who were passing by talked about how they expected to cover five miles that day. That seemed impossible to me. How could anyone jog five miles without stopping?

After about a year my jogging was improving and it seemed to me that maybe I could do a little better if I improved my upper body strength. I started doing chin-ups. Chin-ups were the only upper body strength exercise I used at that time. They were quite easy to do and gave me the impression that I was building body strength. The chin-ups also gave me something to do while waiting for my body to stop perspiring. It was easy to increase the chin-ups to twenty-five or thirty at a time. This was the beginning of adding resistance exercise to my routine.

The area of the Y that had the arrangement set up to do chin-ups had many other pieces of exercise equipment. As I was cooling down, I'd watch others use the weights and do other exercises. One young man was doing push-ups, which continued for a long time. After he finished he came over to me and with a glowing face and broad smile told me how proud he was because he'd just finished doing a set of two hundred push-ups. Not bad!

I remember that during the early part of the summer in 1969, the second year after I started jogging, I got up one Sunday morning and drove over to the South Salem High School track and jogged around the track eight times without stopping. I pushed myself as hard as I could go and made the distance in about eighteen minutes. I got back into the car and drove home. My body was really perspiring and the car seat was soaked when I arrived home. I washed the car seat and took a shower. I was still perspiring after the shower. It usually took about twenty to thirty minutes for the perspiration to stop, but this time it took much longer.

I jogged at the Y three times during the next week and went back to the high school track the following Sunday. This time I took a couple of towels to absorb the sweat when I got back into the car. I covered the seat and seat back with the towels and drove home. The towels were so wet that I could wring them out when I arrived home. I went to the high school track every Sunday for the rest of the summer in addition to my three days at the Y. It rains a lot during the winter in Salem, so my outside jogging was confined to the summer. My time was down to sixteen minutes for two miles by the end of the summer, which was at the end of two years. Two years had gone by and I could now meet Dr. Cooper's test for a man my age.

I found that it was better for my jogging if I waited about three to four hours after eating before I jogged. The several times I did jog soon after eating caused me to become nauseated. So, I have always jogged (except for the learning curve) just before eating a meal. Why? Because the time between meals is usually about four hours, except for breakfast. So, I would jog just before breakfast, lunch, or dinner. This meant that I would eat nothing for those three to four hours. And eating soon after exercising helps me digest the food. It also meant that I soon took absolute control over my eating habits. I began to time my eating habits which caused me to become very aware of when and what food went into my body. My eating habits and diet reached my conscious level. This was the primary step in taking control of my weight. Eventually, I took control of everything that goes into my body. In 1969, after two years, my weight was down to 190 pounds.

In 1969, our daughter, Wendy graduated from South Salem High School and entered the University of Oregon in Eugene. I was thirty-eight years old.

I did some traveling and jogged on my regular days when I was out of town. I would find a high school track and jog around the track. Then one day in late summer of 1969 I went to Butte, Montana, on a business trip and jogged at the Y. Salem's elevation is just a little above sea level, but Butte's elevation is 5,765 feet. Butte is a mining town with some of the town built over a mine. It's a small town filled with dust from the mine and where winter shows up early in September. Butte had a small YMCA and the track was above the basketball court. The track had a steep bank which meant a person must jog at a steady speed to keep from falling off the track. There was no clock near the track and no one at the Y had ever measured the length of the track. So, I jogged until I was tired and then quit. There was no way for me to determine my time and distance. I then went to Helena, Montana, elevation 4,155 feet, and jogged on a high school track. This high school track was the same distance as most high school tracks, one-fourth mile. Even though the elevation is high the town sits on a plateau. Helena is the capital of Montana and a very pretty town. The town was neat and clean. The residents were obviously proud of their location and existence. The residents of Montana are much like the residents of Oregon, as I later learned.

It was at Helena that I found out how much difference altitude makes. It was not possible for me to jog two miles in sixteen minutes. Just jogging the two miles took every ounce of energy in my body. I slowed down considerably after the first mile. It took me twenty minutes to cover the two miles. The person who was with me at the time told me that he could see me slow down and he wondered if I would be able to finish the two miles. My whole body ached, especially my legs, arms, and lungs. It took me several hours to recover. When I returned to Salem, I was able to cover the two miles in sixteen minutes with much less pain. The altitude made a tremendous difference in my time and the energy that it took out of my body.

Now I was beginning to feel healthy and felt like I was taking command of my body. It is and was a great feeling. My routine became pretty well settled by the end of 1970. My jogging time kept lowering slightly for each mile and the amount of energy expended for each jog continued to decrease. The days of dread and exhaustion were now behind me and I began to look forward to my exercise program. By the end of 1970 I felt like jogging had become part of my normal life.

In December 1970 I moved to Anderson, Indiana. I was forty years old. My wife and family joined me in June 1971. Wendy remained in Eugene, Oregon, as a student at the university. Anderson is located about thirty-five miles northeast of Indianapolis. The White River flows through the middle of town. Anderson had a population of about 65,000 people. The elevation is close to sea level, similar to the elevation in Salem. Anderson was kind of a nondescript town with an old city center and one seven story tall new building. General Motors was the major employer and the majority of employees were members of a union. The total GM employment was about 33,000 when we first moved to Anderson. Many of the employees were farmers. Most farms in Indiana raise corn and soybeans, plus a few pigs and hogs. It rains on a regular schedule in the summer in Indiana almost every year, two or three times a week. The crops grow on a regular schedule. The farmers plant the seeds in the spring and harvest the crops in the fall. The farms have been passed down from father to son or daughter for generations, which reduced the average size of the farms to about 100 acres. If the farmers had more than one child, they would divide the farm at death and let the children inherit equally. The family farmers would keep their land, sharecrop, and work for GM. Many of the city residents would go to college, obtain a bachelors degree, then return to GM as a line employee. In 1971 the average earnings for a GM union worker was about $35,000. Husband and wife would both work at the factories, which gave them an excellent standard of living.

Anderson had an excellent YMCA in the downtown section and it was well managed. There was a Big Boy Restaurant on one corner of the block and across the street from the restaurant was the library. I could use the Y, get breakfast or lunch, and spend a half hour or so at the restaurant on most days. So I joined the Y. The jogging track at the Y was located above the basketball court. The track was about five feet wide and slanted towards the inside. The general consensus of opinion was that the track measured twenty-seven laps to a mile.

During the first year after I moved to Anderson I traveled around the state of Indiana nearly every week. Indiana is a provincial state filled with small towns. Indianapolis was originally a railroad hub. The railroad extends from Chicago to Indianapolis, then southeast to Cincinnati, and northeast to Cleveland. It also extends southwest to St. Louis. The trains were long, 150 to 250 cars to a freight train. One man I knew pulled up to a crossing in the evening while a train was passing, fell asleep, and woke up the next morning.

Each week I would be in a different town and use whatever facilities happened to be nearby. Some of the towns had a Y, but usually I found it necessary to travel thirty or forty miles to a larger community to use the Y or other spa facilities. One of the Y's had a small cement outside oval track that was used for jogging. The track was so small that it took about fifty laps to travel one mile. The manager told me that very few people ever came there to jog. On one occasion I went to East Chicago, Indiana, to use the Y. This facility had a track in the upper part of the building with air conditioning vents hanging down over the track. I had to duck under the vents four times in each lap. Another Y in a different town in Indiana had the track in the basement. The heating vents hung over that track so close to the ground that even a midget would have difficulty using it. But the track at the Y in Fort Wayne was really outstanding. In fact, the entire Y facility was superb. I would usually arrive in Fort Wayne around 10 or 11 PM when few people were present, and I had the facility pretty much to myself. It was great, I really enjoyed it. The variety of jogging facilities in the different cities and towns in Indiana really tested my commitment.

I always returned to Anderson on Fridays during 1971 and the Anderson Y became reliable for comparing the time for my miles. The Y and the track were popular and served as a meeting place for many of the citizens. The management was always trying to improve the facility and they tried to include the community and the YMCA users in their decisions. In 1972, they installed a cushioned jogging floor to save wear and tear on the joggers' ankles and legs. But most of the joggers had different opinions about which direction was best for jogging, whether the direction should change on different days of the week, whether those who walk should walk on the outside of the track, or if the walkers should be on the inside of the track.

In 1972, Wendy married Mr. Douglas Edward Sabin in Eugene, Oregon. They took a year off to work and save some money even though they were both students at the University of Oregon. I was forty-one years old. I was still doing chin-ups and had built the number up to seventy-five. I went into the weight room of the Y to do the chin-ups from a high bar after jogging.

I met Merle Kelly while living in Anderson and jogging at the Y. He was a weight lifting champion and an international weight lifting referee. He weighed about 154 pounds and had been the nation's weight lifting champion in his class for several years before I met him. He was my age (41) and had been lifting weights since he was 15. His body was in perfect shape.

Merle Kelly was normally in the weight room when I arrived. He worked for General Motors and his shift coincided with my regular schedule. One day in 1973, a new member of the Y came in, tried using the bench press, and asked Merle what he should do to create a physique like Merle's. Merle's response to him was "just do whatever you want to do." Later, after the gentleman had left, I asked Merle why he didn't give the man a more complete answer. Merle said several hundred people had come into the gym over the last few years and had asked the same question. He said he used to give them instructions, but after a couple of weeks they would stop coming in. They seemed to believe they could accomplish in a couple of weeks the same results Merle had achieved during the last twenty-five years. When they found that work was involved, they would quit. Merle said that when someone comes in, works out, and is still at it after three or four weeks, then he'll give him all the assistance and advice he could use.

One day a man came into the weight room and attempted to bench press 135 pounds. He couldn't get the bar off his chest. Merle asked me to lift one end of the bar while he lifted the other. I couldn't do it. My chin-ups were of no value from a standpoint of strength. I switched to lifting weights and began with 95 pounds at the bench press. I later began doing curls with the weights, starting with 45 pounds for the total weight for both arms. I also started doing squats using very light weights. I found that using the weights after jogging gave my body the same chance to cool down as doing chin-ups. I would spend about forty-five minutes using the weights and doing the other exercises, and by that time my body was cool enough to shower. I started doing sit-ups at the same time. At first I would lay on the floor and do ten sit-ups. Then I gradually increased to twenty-five sit-ups, and I started to use an incline board to increase the stress on my stomach muscles.

When I began jogging I thought it would take five years to correct my health. My concern was to use my speed as the monitor, continually improve, and when I'd reach the goal of jogging two miles under sixteen minutes time and I had also jogged for five years, then I could quit jogging. Well, a funny thing happened on the way to the opera, I had developed a habit. After the five years were over, I could start to pay attention to other events relating to jogging, not just my time.

By 1973 my jogging became a standard routine, even though the hours and locations changed, my routine never changed. My breathing during the jog set into a pattern. During the first quarter mile, it would build up to a steady, heavier respiration and stay at the same level for the balance of the jog. (Since 1973 there has almost always been enough lung and leg power to speed up the jog during the last sixteenth mile.) My jogging time was a consistent 7'30" per mile for two miles. Occasionally, I'd jog a little farther. I'd add a quarter mile or one half mile extra from time to time. One day in that year I experienced what is referred to as a "runner's high." I felt a sense of euphoria and ease during the second mile. It felt like jogging was as natural as walking. So, I continued jogging for four miles and never tired. I have felt this "runner's high" only one other time during the thirty-seven years I've been jogging.

Also in 1973, the Anderson Y had a big clock placed at one end of the track with a large second hand that made it easy to time the laps. I found that it became easier to increase my speed at a steady pace by covering each lap in the same number of seconds. I could easily jog each lap in seventeen seconds and complete the two miles under sixteen minutes. The clock made it easy to reduce my time. I would knock off one second every three laps and reduce my time by eighteen seconds over the two miles. I used this technique for the next several years and after about eight years of jogging my speed had increased to 7'15" per mile. I could never cover the two miles any faster than that. By now my weight was down to 175 pounds.

During the 1970s, people would do strange things on the jogging tracks. Sometimes people would try to jog backwards, backside first and against the flow of the other joggers. They had to turn their heads from side to side to try to see where they were going. If the direction of the joggers was counterclockwise, the backwards joggers would try to jog clockwise. They were very, very slow. Talk about confusion. The backward joggers didn't seem to understand why they were causing a problem. I asked a couple of them what they were trying to accomplish and the response was that jogging backwards would help them in their daily lives. It never made any sense to me since I've never seen anyone going about their daily lives walking backwards. This peculiarity seemed to be confined to Indiana, at least in my experience. The Y management finally invited all joggers to become members of a committee to establish the jogging rules. About fifteen joggers agreed to form the committee. The committee met five or six times and developed a set of jogging rules that attempted to satisfy all of those who used the track. It worked out quite well.

Once a year the Anderson Y would clean and repair the facilities, which meant the track was closed for a week. I would usually go to the Muncie, Indiana, Y during that week. The Muncie track was larger, and it took fewer revolutions to complete a mile. Some of the joggers in Muncie would travel counterclockwise, while at the same time others would travel clockwise. The track was seldom full of joggers as a result of this procedure. The only way I could cope with it was to jog far on the outside of the track and be prepared to stop at any moment. If two people jogging in opposite directions were to meet head on it would cause quite a collision.

I had regular medical examinations every six months after I started jogging and I've taken thyroid medication for an underactive thyroid every day since I was twenty-five years old. My physician in Anderson, Dr. Rosenbaum, would require me to come to his office every three months for a regular exam before renewing the prescription. He'd administer a blood test, check my blood pressure, height, and weight. In 1973 my blood pressure averaged 120/80. My heartbeat rate was around 70 bpm. My average weight was 175, but Dr. Rosenbaum found that my weight fluctuated by two pounds between summer and winter. I weighed two pounds more in the winter than summer. My weight remained the same for eight years with the two pound fluctuation. And all of my other vital signs remained within the same ranges. Physically, I felt great.

In 1974 Cindy graduated from Madison Heights High School in Anderson and entered Purdue University. Wendy and Doug graduated from the University of Oregon. Wendy and Doug found jobs and soon bought a small house in Eugene that became their home for many years. I was forty-three years old.

Since my jogging routine was firmly established, I began to concentrate on my resistance exercises. I gradually increased the pounds I could lift when using the weights. I would use the weights for curls without feeling psychological pressure to increase the pounds. The bench press became the biggest challenge for me. I stopped doing the squats, and clean and jerk, because I believed my legs got enough exercise with the jogging. I decided the curls, bench press, and sit-ups, would give me good body tone. Most of the serious weight lifters concentrated on the bench press, squats, and clean and jerk. Some of the weight lifters would load 300 to 350 pounds on those bars, and there was no way I could compete with them. I was trying to build up to 150 pounds and those big fellows just didn't like to take the weights off the bars for my turn to lift and then put the weights back on. So, I had to change my time schedule to allow me to be in the weight room when they were somewhere else.

By 1975 I was bench pressing 150 pounds and curling 75 pounds. I'd go into a different room to do the sit-ups, a room which had a boxer's punching bag. I put a board on a thirty-degree incline and would do thirty-five sit-ups. For about a year, one young man would come into that room to practice boxing. He was preparing to enter a boxing tournament. He became very proficient and although he won several matches he decided to give up boxing. When I asked him why he was quitting, he said his wife was opposed to him entering the ring with the chance of being permanently harmed. I think he made a wise choice.

By 1976, I was bench pressing 175 pounds and was curling 90 pounds. I didn't just lay on the bench and press 175 pounds, I'd always press less weight several times before pressing the maximum weight. For example, I would press 135 pounds 10 times. Then 155 pounds 10 times. And then

170 pounds 2, 3, or 4 times. When I moved up from 170 pounds to 175 pounds, I'd press the 175 pounds once the first time. Then I'd build up my ability to lift it three or four times. I'd keep working on the higher weight until it felt comfortable to press more than just one or two times. The curls stayed about the same and the sit-ups were the same.

It can get cold in Indiana in the winter. I've seen it get to –17° F, and it was much colder with the wind chill factored in. We lived in a townhouse apartment, and one day the snow blew through the seal of the sliding doors and formed a tapered line across our living room floor. During the winter of 1977, the snow was so deep it completely covered outside the first floor of our apartment. Our bedroom was on the second floor, and Leslie's cat would walk out our bedroom window to do his business outside. We dug a small cave in the snow by the sliding doors in the living room on the first floor so our poodle could get outside. On another winter day I was driving from Fort Wayne to Anderson, and I could see sheets of ice about two feet thick that spanned the highway and about 300 or 400 feet on both sides of the road. It is very unlikely that many people will exercise outdoors in weather like this. So, some areas really need indoor facilities.

In 1977, I was forty-six years old, and Leslie graduated from Madison Heights High School. She and a friend, Bonita Skelton, decided to move to Florida. Leslie took all of her money out of her savings account, her friend bought a used car, they both packed their clothes and other belongings and away they went. She lived in Florida for about two and one-half years. She returned to Anderson in the fall of 1980.

During 1977 a man came into the weight room to work out. He knew what he was doing, but it was obvious that he was out of shape. He came in every day and established a regular routine. Within a month he had worked his body into reasonably good condition. I asked him about his goal. He told me that he was the United States Kickboxing Champion in his class and that he was preparing for a championship match that was to take place in two more months. He stayed with his routine for the next two months and formed his body into what looked to me to be perfect condition. It was amazing to me how he had control over the outcome and how well he knew his time frame for preparation for the bout. He won the bout and retained his championship. At that time, Kickboxing was a relatively new sport, and the city of Anderson didn't realize a national champion lived there.

Trying to meet the same time and distance goal and exact jogging schedule began to produce some negative results. I would pull a muscle. Then I had to find a method of soothing the muscles and still jog. When I pulled a muscle I would first apply heat. That made it worse. Then I applied cold. The cold helped reduce the muscle soreness much better than heat. Then I tried binding the sore muscle with elastic cloth tape while I jogged. Whether I used cold or tape, it would take several weeks for the sore muscle to be repaired. Over time, I think I've tried just about every pain reduction method known to man.

The most severe pain I encountered was a torn Achilles tendon. I tore it in 1978, my eleventh year of jogging, while living in Anderson. I decided to not allow the injury to prevent me from exercising. I bought a long cloth-elastic bandage and wrapped my foot and leg from the toes up to the top of my calf so tightly that I couldn't move my ankle. Then I'd put on my shoes and jog two miles around the track. It was a very slow jog, but my object was to manage my cardiovascular system, and even a slow jog was better than none at all. This routine lasted for seven months. *One day during my jog I felt no pain in my tendon, leg, or foot, so I stopped and removed the bandage and tried jogging without it. The pain was gone. The tendon was healed.* Over the next several weeks, I increased my speed back up to my old time, before the injury, of 7'30" per mile for the two miles.

In 1978 Cindy graduated from Purdue University, Phi Beta Kappa, and married her college companion, Lawrence Gregg Fitzgerald. They moved to Dayton, Ohio, where Cindy entered the University of Dayton to begin work on her master's program. I was forty-seven years old. Cindy and Gregg divorced in 1979.

In 1979 a man came into the weight lifting area in the Y and began his routine. He had a muscular body and it appeared as though he had lifted weights in the past. Over time, he increased the amount of weights he was lifting too rapidly. A couple of months later he damaged several muscles in his body while bench pressing. Other members of the Y had to lift the weights off his body and carry him out of the gym. I never saw him again. His results served as a permanent reminder to me that I must know my capacity with the weights.

By 1979 my maximum bench press was 195 pounds. I really wasn't interested in increasing the amount of weight I used for the curls, so I was still doing the curls with 90 pounds of weight. My sit-ups were still at thirty-five, which was sufficient for my purposes.

In 1980, my wife, Dorothy, had suffered enough with the problems we experienced in Indiana, and she decided to move back to Salt Lake City, Utah. I was involved in a series of lawsuits over work related issues. The lawsuits were anxiety provoking for the entire family. The lawsuits lasted for fourteen years from 1971 through 1985. I encountered serious issues of trust with most of my attorneys. Two of the suits were against former attorneys. My primary lawsuits were filed against an insurance company I had worked for, with the insurance company president as a codefendant in one action. The insurance company president engaged in extortion with one of the judges. (The judge, Michael T. Dugan of Indianapolis, was sentenced to 17 years in prison on July 5, 1989, for demanding and accepting bribes from a number of people.)[1] Deception and betrayal of this nature caused serious emotional problems in my family. My exercising was a key to maintaining my health and stability throughout the ordeal. But Dorothy just didn't want to deal with it anymore. Dorothy found work in Salt Lake City, rented an apartment, and remained there until 1986.

Cindy obtained her master's degree at the University of Dayton.

In 1980, I began to experiment with other jogging distances beyond two miles. Once, I jogged for five miles. But most of the time it was between two and three miles. I set my new goal at twenty minutes, instead of two miles. By now, a twenty-minute jog was easy. In fact, if someone

---

1. United States of America v. Michael T. Dugan, II, Southern District of Indiana, Indianapolis Division. Cause No. IP88-78-CR. Jury verdict returned 5-26-89, guilty on a variety of charges of bribery and extortion, including a true bill of unlawfully obtaining money from James Eckman, President of First Equity Security Life Insurance Company.

was jogging a little faster than me, I could use him as a draft and increase my speed for a mile or so. I had reached an exercise level of satisfaction and just continued the same routine for the next several years.

In 1980 and 1981, I gradually increased my bench press maximum weight to two hundred pounds. My other resistance exercises remained the same. I was quite satisfied with my body tone. My only challenge was to see how much weight I could bench press without damaging my body.

When I was forty-nine years old, in 1980, my sister, Ruth, arranged a family reunion. I hadn't seen some of my siblings in many years and didn't recognize most of them. I wouldn't have known some of my brothers and sisters if I'd passed them on the street. It took all day to get reacquainted. Ruth had an excellent idea, and it brought the family much closer together. Ruth passed away on October 26, 1981, at age fifty-three. She suffered from leukemia and had kept the illness secret from the rest of her siblings. She knew she had leukemia for several years before her death and wanted to be able to see everyone before she passed away. That was the principal reason she had arranged the family reunion.

In 1981, I was fifty years old. Leslie moved to Salt Lake City to be near her mother.

In, 1982 Leslie married Jeffry Morrison.

My brother David passed away on July 25, 1982. He suffered from multiple myeloma for several years before his death. Multiple myeloma is a particularly painful form of cancer that eats away at the victim's bones. I was fifty-one years old.

I moved to Indianapolis in February 1983. I located a spa close to my apartment and joined the first day I moved into town. Actually, I lived in the town of Speedway, which is part of Indianapolis. Speedway is where the Indianapolis 500 auto race is run each May, and I lived right across the street from the racetrack. I never went to a race, but once I did watch the police direct traffic to and from the racetrack. They had the traffic pattern so well organized that it only took about two hours for all of the drivers to arrive, park and enter the speedway. And it took less time for them to leave.

The Indianapolis spa kept the temperature at sixty degrees all year around. The track was very small, but with the temperature set at sixty degrees it was easy to maintain a fluid jog for a longer distance. I would jog for a steady twenty-four minutes three times a week. Then I'd use the weights and spend time engaged in pleasant conversation with other members of the spa. Quite a few members were Indianapolis policemen. They kept their bodies in excellent physical condition, and they were perfect gentlemen. Some of their wives would work out at the same time. It was an excellent arrangement for the families.

Most spas have weight rooms with a variety of free weights and bars that hold the weights. Today most facilities have a variety of machines and gadgets with pulleys. They all seem to have treadmills. Jogging on treadmills is fine once a person gets used to them. The difference is that a treadmill has a moving floor, whereas when jogging on a track or outdoors I'm jogging on a stationary floor. I feel more in control if the floor is stationary.

I tried jogging four, five, and six, days a week from 1981 to 1983 while I lived in Anderson and when I first moved to Indianapolis. Four days a week seemed to be okay, but five and six days seemed to exhaust my body so much that I wasn't really refreshed the next time I went for my jog. I was discussing this with another jogger at the spa in Indianapolis, and he told me that studies had shown the body needs about thirty-six hours of rest between workouts. Then I tried jogging every other day. Jogging every other day worked out just fine from the point of view of refreshing my body, but the routine caused me to keep track of each jogging day. I would forget whether or not I had jogged the day before. I changed my routine again to jog three times a week. Jogging three times a week meant I could select three days as my jogging days and little memory work was involved. For several years I would jog on Monday, Wednesday, and Friday. I eventually changed the schedule to Tuesday, Thursday, and Sunday. I changed it again to Tuesday, Thursday, and Saturday. The Tuesday, Thursday, and Saturday or Sunday, schedule meant I had three full days of work with only two days of jogging interfering with my work schedule.

In 1983 Wendy and Doug Sabin became the parents of Robert Edward. I was fifty-three years old.

In 1984 Leslie and Jeffry Morrison became the parents of Angela Brooke.

Most spas like to play music to entertain the members. It was at the Indianapolis spa where I heard the song "Staying Alive" by the Bee Gees. It sounded to me like they were singing "Har, har, har, har, staying alive, staying alive." Those are the words I remember, and those are the words that go through my mind many times while I'm jogging. I'd bring those words to my mind and repeat them silently, especially when the jog was tough. "Har, har, har, har, staying alive, staying alive. That's why I'm doing this, to stay alive, staying alive." Those words became a hook for me, if I needed a hook.

One of the members of the Indianapolis spa had very poor eyesight. He was nearsighted, and he had heard about a new operation which could correct nearsightedness. He elected to have the operation, but for him, it was a failure. He lost his vision entirely. Those operations have been perfected so that they are now nearly failsafe, but for him it was a tragedy. Even so, he continued to exercise at the spa until his blindness made in impossible for him to continue without personal assistance.

Another member of the spa was training for a marathon. He was heavier than most runners, but he continued to train for several months and he did run the marathon. The week following the marathon he came into the spa and jogged for about five miles. He was totally exhausted at the end. The next week he was back, but he found he could only jog about one-and-a-half miles. He complained about soreness of muscles throughout his body. I never saw him again. A young married couple came to the spa and jogged on a regular basis. She became pregnant, but they continued to jog together. They both jogged up until about three days before she gave birth to their child. Parenting took over, and they never returned. Two brothers came into the spa every night after work. They were bricklayers and told me that when they worked out at the spa at night it made their bricklaying duties much easier during the day. Their theory was that the bricks were very light compared to the weights they used in the spa.

A different member of the Indianapolis spa would jog two miles outside all year around. He was about thirty years old and in good condition. I asked him if he didn't get cold during the middle of the winter. He answered that he was jogging too fast to let the temperature bother him. He was only gone for ten or eleven minutes. The key here is that under most conditions a person can exercise regardless of the weather. Sometimes the weather makes it impossible and indoor facilities are preferred, but a person can still find a way to get the exercising in.

I lived in Indiana for fifteen years, and I was in sales all of those years. I traveled a lot and my hours were unpredictable. There were days when I finished before noon, days I'd finish at 6:00 PM, and days when I finished at midnight. When I traveled, it wasn't possible for me to jog on a regular schedule. Sometimes I'd jog at noon other times at 6 PM. There were times that I jogged at 10 PM or midnight. I've jogged at every hour of a 24-hour day. Some of the Y's and spas remained open 24-hours each day. It gets very hot and humid in Indiana during the summertime. A person could start perspiring just thinking about exercising during the daytime. Some days during the summer the temperature would get no lower than sixty-five or seventy degrees. Add that to the humidity, and jogging without air conditioning was terrible. It was easier for me to get up at 4, 5, or 6 AM and complete my exercise at that time. I wasn't alone, there were usually six or seven other joggers at the Y doing the same thing.

In January 1986, I moved to Santa Clara, California. I was fifty-five years old. The San Francisco Bay branches off into two directions, East and South. Santa Clara and San Jose are on the south end of the bay. This area is known as Silicon Valley. Both cities are in Santa Clara County, as are Campbell, Sunnyvale, Cupertino, Palo Alto, and several other cities. This is a large urban area. The entire Bay is populated by about 5.5 million people. Many of the people in Silicon Valley like to play tennis, swim, and do other exercises in the open air. The weather is more in tune to outdoor activities year around.

I found no inside jogging tracks in the San Jose area. That meant that I would be jogging outside for the next few years. First, I found several high schools with oval tracks and began jogging around the tracks when school wasn't in session. The tracks became muddy when it rained, and it rained a lot during the first several months I was in California. So, when it rained, I would jog around the streets in the neighborhood of my apartment and then do push-ups and other exercises at the apartment. After a couple of weeks, I joined a 24-Hour Fitness Center on Hillsdale Avenue in San Jose and used those facilities for my weights and body tone exercises. I could now bench press about 215 pounds. My curl weights were up to about 100 pounds, and I used machines where I could push weights with my legs without squatting. I added dips with my arms using one of the pieces of equipment at the center.

Dorothy moved back with me in the summer of 1986 and we both moved to a condo in Santa Clara. The Fitness Center was a long drive from our condo and my office, which meant taking extra time out of the day. I found there was an excellent exercise facility near my apartment and closer to my office and our condo. It was the Decathlon Club in Santa Clara. It is really an outstanding facility. The club is situated near Highway 101. It's located in the midst of many Silicon Valley businesses.

The Decathlon Club became my base for using the weights, showering, and changing clothes. I'd usually exercise just before lunch. I'd put on my jogging clothes and jog along several streets, over Highway 101 on a ramp, three times around Mission College, and come back over the freeway to the health club. Sometimes I'd jog around different blocks to and from the freeway overpass. The total distance was close to four miles. The jogging time was averaging about 7'30" per mile. But it wasn't possible to get an exact measurement of the distance. After my jog, I'd use the weights at the club. I built my bench press maximum weight to 225 pounds. I had developed a routine with the weights and resistance machine to exercise most of my upper body. I was doing bench presses, arm curls, push-ups, leg presses (not upper body), and sit-ups. (Eventually I dropped the sit-ups because of hemorrhoid problems.) The exercise routine took about two hours from beginning to end. For me, the weights and upper body exercises were for body tone, and I didn't consider them as part of my cardiovascular exercise. However, studies now show weight training to be an excellent cardiovascular exercise. I think using the weights have been helpful for me.

In early 1987, I was bench pressing 225 pounds without a spotter. My left arm collapsed and the bar fell down across my throat with the left side of the bar touching the floor, the middle of the bar on my throat, and the right side of the bar was still up in the air held by my right arm. It damaged my throat and made it difficult for me to talk. I had a business appointment in Livermore, California, about an hour's drive away. I drove to Livermore and made an appointment with a doctor preceding my business appointment. The doctor was delighted to see the damage because it was so unusual. She asked if she could take pictures of it before beginning treatment. I had no objection, but it turned out she didn't have her camera in the office. There wasn't much she could do in any event and she advised me to allow it to heal itself, which it did.

In the summer of 1987 it was becoming more difficult to jog three times around Mission College, breathing became more difficult so I cut the distance to twice around the college. Sometimes when I'd get back to the rise of the freeway overpass, I'd have to stop jogging and walk up the incline. Then I could start jogging again on the downhill side. It seemed to me that I was just getting older which made it harder to jog. By now I was fifty-six years old.

In September 1987, Dorothy and I bought a home and moved to San Jose. It was too far away from the Decathlon Club, so I rejoined the 24-Hour Fitness club, which was about twenty minutes away from our home. I would jog two miles around the neighborhood three times a week and then go to the club to do the resistance exercising (weights, etc.). I changed my jogging time to early morning. I'd jog at 6:00 AM then go to the club, exercise, shower, dress, and go to work.

In 1988 Wendy and Doug became the parents of Rachel Marie, and Leslie and Jeff became the parents of Anastasia (Stacey) Marie. I was fifty-seven years old.

In 1988, twenty-one years after beginning my exercise routine, and eighteen years after the end of my predicted life span, I could really feel myself slowing down. I found it more and more difficult to keep up my speed so I increased my distance. I'd jog from our home on Walnut Blossom Drive, north to Hayes, jog right and north again on Apple Blossom

Drive, west on Chenowyth to Cherry Blossom, Guava Blossom, Prune Blossom, Pear Blossom, to Lean, south on Lean to Lime Blossom, Cashew Blossom, the other end of Cherry Blossom, across Lean and south to Hayes (Lean to Hayes curves east and there is a lot of traffic. It was necessary to dodge the cars nearly every morning.), west to Eagles, south to Blossom Hill Road (around Oak Grove High School), east across Lean, across Walnut Blossom, past Town & Country mobile home community, and on to Beswick, then to the Cottle Road-Hayes intersection, west on Hayes to Walnut Blossom, and home. This is 3.15 miles.

There are many intersections where I had to compete with cars. The Beswick intersection is well lit at night. There are quite a few street lights, plus the lights of the all-night Chevron station. The north side of Blossom Hill at Beswick is the main entrance and exit to the Magic Sands mobile home community. This intersection is dangerous because the cars leave the mobile home community with the drivers looking east (their left) to spot oncoming traffic if they plan to turn right (west). They always drive into the pedestrian lane and seldom look right for a pedestrian. Going around the Cottle Road-Hayes intersection and turning west on Hayes is the back entrance to the same mobile home community. A fence blocks the view for cars leaving the community so the drivers can't see a pedestrian until the car is on the sidewalk. This is another danger point. In most areas of California outdoor jogging is the only option. So, I needed to find a route that would be very familiar to me.

Back to my breathing problem. From time to time, I was so out of breath that I had to stop and walk before continuing my jog. It got to the point where I could only jog a mile without stopping. One morning in December 1988, I'd reached the corner of Chenowyth and Lean, I had jogged about one-half mile and had to sit down. I was completely out of breath. I sat on the curb for ten to fifteen minutes without the strength to get up. I finally told myself that I must get back to the house. I forced myself to get to my feet and gingerly walked back to the house. I sat at the breakfast table drinking coffee for a few minutes and finally decided to call a doctor. My internist, Dr. Richard Adrouny, asked me to come right in to his office. He completed an ECG and found irregularities. He had me admitted to Kaiser Hospital on Cottle Road and asked Dr. Joseph Casey, a cardiologist, to perform an angiogram. Dr. Casey found an artery to be 90 percent blocked. I was transferred to Good Samaritan Hospital because I was not a member of the Kaiser medical plan. Dr. Casey then performed angioplasty and I was released from the hospital. I was hospitalized for about four days.

After I returned home, I stayed in bed for a day, then I wanted to get out and jog again. So, the next day I jogged the regular three miles a little slower than usual and I suffered no adverse effects. I immediately got back into my regular routine and quickly built my time back up to the eight minute mile. Three months later, in March 1989, I was at 24-Hour Fitness, doing leg presses, when I felt a severe pain in my chest and felt faint. I stood up and was trying to control my equilibrium when an acquaintance, a preacher, began to explain the presence of God. I remember thinking, "I'm closer to God than you might suspect." I went home, called Dr. Casey, and explained what happened. He asked me to come right in to his office. He determined I had a heart attack. He assumed the first angioplasty had failed. He did another angiogram and found a different artery was blocked. He performed another angioplasty which was successful. I was out of commission for about four or five days this time.

A nurse at Good Samaritan Hospital in San Jose told me to never eat fat again. She said to cut even the smallest amount of fat from meat that I eat. I decided to eat only chicken, turkey, and fish. Two days after returning home I was back jogging, only slower than before. My wife, Dorothy, would get out of bed and sit by the living room window watching to see if I'd return. When I did return, she'd go back to bed. This continued for about six months.

I decided to set up my resistance exercises at home. I had a bench made out of a 6"× 10"× 95" block of wood set upon two cinder blocks at each end. I bought a mat and some free weights so that each hand would work independently of the other. The weights allow me to arrange any number of pounds to do a variety of curls and bench lifts. Now if an arm collapses, the weight will just fall to the ground from one arm because each arm presses a separate weight. First, I would do two sets of curls, 10 reps each, using 25 pounds on each arm. Then I'd do four sets of curls, 10 reps each, using 40 pounds on each arm. I used 70 pounds in each arm to do bench presses. I'd do three sets of 24, 22, and 20 repetitions. After doing the bench presses, I'd do a set of 45 dips from the bench. I bought a set of aluminum "power bars" to do push-ups to replace the sit-ups. It took me a few months to develop skills with the push-ups. Dorothy would tell me that I was doing "head bobs." I kept at it, and after a year I could do 60 push-ups without too much difficulty. By this time my weight was down to 171 pounds.

In 1990 Cindy married Daniel Warren Campbell. Dan lived in southern California, but was transferred to the San Jose area soon after their marriage. They bought a home in Campbell and settled down. I was fifty-nine years old.

That same year my mother gave me a journal. I had no other use for the journal, so I decided to keep a log of my jogs. Up until this time I only kept the record in my head but with the experience of the heart attacks, it seemed to me that I could spot the occurrence of a serious medical problem by writing down my time, distance, and comments, and then make comparisons over the months and years. On March 30, 1991, I began keeping a log of my jogging. On that day my distance was 3.15 miles and my time was 27'57". My next entry was on April 20, 1991, and my time was 29'23". Thereafter, I recorded each time I jogged. I also recorded heart and money problems, plus a comment. In 1991 my recorded time would range between 27 and 29 minutes for the 3.15 miles. Once a week I would jog an extra one and seven tenths miles, but I didn't time the extra jog. By now I was sixty years old and in my twenty-third year of jogging, and I had experienced two angioplasty operations and one or two heart attacks. I'm not sure if the first event was a heart attack or simply artery blockage. Dr. Casey treated it as a heart attack. My time was averaging about nine minutes per mile, my weight was between 170 and 172 pounds, and my blood pressure was still 120/80. The time of each jog was different, the difference being as little as one second and as much as two-and-a-half minutes for the 3.15 miles. Usually my time would fluctuate up or down one minute plus several seconds. My notes reflect that some of the time the first half of the jog was easy and the last half hard, and other times it was the reverse. The occasions when the entire jog seemed easy and smooth were few and far between.

In 1991 I changed cardiologists from Dr. Casey to Dr. Jack Siegel because my medical insurance plan excluded Dr. Casey's medical group. I settled into a long term routine. I wake up at 5:30 AM, I use the bathroom, weigh myself and put on my exercise clothes. Then I exercise my neck by turning it back and forth ten times. (Our necks can become sore and brittle if not exercised.) I twist my upper torso ten times to loosen the back muscles. Next I lean on the kitchen counter and bend my back forward and back again ten times. I do ten knee bends. Then I spread my feet far apart and touch my right fingers to my left toes, then my left fingers to my right toes. I do this a total of twenty-five times with each arm. After the toe touch I stretch one leg out in front and one leg in back and rock back and forth ten times, then I switch legs and repeat. I do these exercises every day. It's a six minute routine.

Before I begin my regular jog, I jog around the block twice. Twice around is a six tenths of a mile. I use the bathroom again. Next, I start and complete my jog. After finishing my jog I always drink a glass of water. It never tastes better than at this time. I water some plants or do other yard work while my body cools down. After the jog and after I've cooled down, I change T-shirts, socks and shoes, put on a pair of gloves and do my resistance exercises.

In 1991 I was taking long jogging strides. It was easy and comfortable to stretch the legs out and just move along. I was back into my stride. But over the next several years I found I was slowing down, so I narrowed my strides to see how it would affect my time. To my amazement, it reduced my time for the distance. I could jog faster. When I switched back to longer strides and tried to keep the same time it really was exhausting. When I shortened my stride again I felt better when the jog was over. (Talking about a long stride, in Eugene, Oregon, in the mid 1990s, I, my son-in-law Doug Sabin, and the two children, were at a park by the Willamette River when a runner came around a curve. He stretched his legs out so that they were horizontal to the ground, a complete split three feet above the ground. That runner was amazing.)

I learned over the years to pay attention to my muscles. It took me about twenty-five years to learn to slow down when I feel a muscle tightening. I now continue at a slower pace until the tightness disappeared, then I move faster again. It took me a long time to understand that it isn't necessary to try to complete the jog at the same speed each time.

I ran with a very small pebble in my shoe one day in 2002. It left a sore on the bottom of my foot, kind of like a callous. I tried treating it myself for about six months, but the callous would peel off and the sore remained. I finally visited Dr. Richard Meltzer, a podiatrist. A cream he asked me to apply required another year to eliminate the callous. Dr. Meltzer said that if the cream didn't work then he could remove the sore with surgery. The cream took a long time to work and I decided against the operation. The sore finally disappeared after several more months.

On January 2, 1992, my time was still 27'54" and my weight was 166 pounds. During the year my weight dropped down to 160 pounds, and my jogging time averaged between 25 and 26 minutes, but there was a difference of as much as 1 minute and 28 seconds between my slowest and fastest jogs. Between January 2, 1993, and May 1, 1993, my time averaged between 25 and 27 minutes and my weight fluctuated between 156 and 160 pounds. After May 1, the time averaged between 26 and 28 minutes. I also tried to change my mental attitude by making notes each time I jogged, commenting that I had had a very good run. I made the same notes clear through 1997. The record shows that my recording the notes made no difference in my time over distance. My mental attitude didn't make much difference, it was how loose or tight my body felt from tension when I began the jog that made the difference. Some people say its how the body flows. Towards the end of 1993, my time increased to an average between 27 and 28 minutes.

My brother, Louis, passed away on January 11, 1993, at age fifty-nine. His second heart attack was fatal. It came suddenly in the night. I was sixty-two years old.

From November 28, 1993, to July 10, 1994, I changed to a vegetarian diet. I wanted to see if taking meat completely out of my diet would help my heart. My theory was that if it did help, my jogging time would reduce, my speed would increase, and my heart would get stronger. It made no difference in my jogging time, but it did make a difference in my strength in handling the weights. It took a lot more energy to handle the weights. In July, I began eating chicken, turkey, and fish again. I've eaten beef maybe once a year since then and I'll eat lean pork chops from time to time. I do what the nurse told me to do, I cut every small piece of fat off the meat and make sure it's cooked well-done. My family complained about my diet for several years because they didn't want to eat my fixed diet and my wife didn't want to fix two different meals. Now it is difficult for them to eat beef. My wife will eat beef at restaurants on occasion, but the grandchildren seldom ask for beef any more, except for fast food hamburgers or cheeseburgers. Angela decided to become a vegetarian, but for different reasons, and that lasted about a year.

On November 28, 1993, I pulled a calf muscle in my leg. This caused my time to increase to 36 minutes for the jog. The next jog was 33 minutes, then 32'39", then 28'26", and several jogs later it was down to between 27 and 28 minutes. During 1994 my time averaged 28 minutes in the winter and 27 minutes in the summer.

In 1994 I was doing 64 push-ups. I also did 12 repetitions with the 25-pound dumbbells of arm curls, first one arm, then the other arm, then 12 repetitions using both arms together. Then I'd use one 25-pound weight to do 12 lifts, which exercised my forearms. Next, using two short bars and 35 pounds attached to each bar, I'd do 12 curls the same as with the 25 pound weights, I'd do additional sets so that it totaled four sets of curls. I'd rest for two minutes between each set. I'd attach 65 pounds of weights on each of the same bars I used for curls, lay down on the pad and press the weights up (like a bench press) for 20 repetitions. I'd rest 4 to 5 minutes. Then I'd do another set with 140 pound weights for 18 repetitions. Then I'd rest 4 to 5 minutes and do a third set of 16 repetitions. Finally I'd do 36 arm dips from the bench with my hands placed in back of me on the bench and my legs straight out in front. The routine was finished. I'd drink a glass of orange juice when using the weights.

Most people decide upon ten reps for any routine using weights or stretches. Why do I use different numbers? I read a book that claimed it was just as easy to multiply by any number other than ten, so I decided to try the process, beginning with my exercises. I wound up doing extra reps in every set, but it never improved my math skills.

My mother passed away on December 19, 1994, at age eighty-eight. She suffered from heart failure, but the cause of death was considered to be natural. My mother lived for forty-three years after the death of my father. She lived half of her life as a widow. After she reached sixty-five, she worked as a caretaker of older persons who needed assistance. She lived mostly alone and provided for herself for the rest of her life. I was sixty-four years old.

On June 18, 1995, my weight was 160, and it's averaged 160 to the date of this book. My weight will fluctuate one to two pounds per week. When it goes up, I drop it back down. When it goes below 160, I bring it back up. I eat less food for several days to lose weight and eat more food for several days to gain weight. That's the only guide I've ever used.

One day in 1995, I was doing push-ups and noticed that my hands and arms seemed to be aligned more to the inside of the power bars, rather than directly over the top of the bars. I decided to realign my hands so the wrists were not bent, but on a straight angle from my hands. The next thing I knew, my left hand slipped off the bar and I fell down on my face, smashing my jaw. It hurt, but nothing was broken. I got back on the power bars and finished the set without worrying about the alignment of my wrists.

On September 10, 1995, I fainted in the bathroom and it took about ten minutes for me to revive. My wife called the paramedics, and they were standing over me when I regained consciousness. They took me to Good Samaritan Hospital for a day, but no cause for fainting could be found. My pulse rate was below 40, so I assumed my fainting was caused by the low pulse rate. I was released from the hospital and returned to my regular routine. After being released from the hospital, my primary physician, Dr. Charles Sheptin, ordered new tests, including a chest X-ray. The technician took the picture and brought it out to the viewing screen, which was next to my chair, along with a second X-ray from another man. I heard the technician say, "Wow, look at this!" I came over and took a look. My lungs were twice as large as the other person's lungs. The many years of jogging increased the size of my lungs. It is my theory that the increased size of my lungs has prevented the onset of emphysema. I had smoked tobacco for twenty years. Other members of my family and some of my friends who smoked several years suffered from emphysema at some point in their lives.

My next jog was September 13. In November I turned sixty-five.

On October 28, 1996, I felt a serious pain in my lower abdomen that lasted four days. I flew to Florida October 29 to visit my brother, Conrad. I was constipated and assumed the pain would disappear when I solved the constipation problem. It didn't. I returned to San Jose and waited until January before seeing Dr. Sheptin. He sent me to a specialist who found I had a hernia. On February 15, 1997, the specialist performed a hernia operation. I walked the distance for the next week, and by February 27, I was back to the regular jogging time of under thirty minutes. Several weeks later my time was around twenty-eight minutes.

On May 1, 1997, our daughter, Leslie, with her two daughters, moved in with my wife and me, because she had separated from her husband. The addition to our household created tension for everyone. I was sixty-six years old.

On May 13, 1997, I pulled a muscle in my back, which was very painful. It isn't possible to wrap my body to relieve any back pain and I still needed to do my exercise. I gritted my teeth and began to jog. Just moving from the walking pace to a slow jog jarred my back and sent shooting pains throughout my body and up to my brain. I kept jogging. The pain slowly receded. As the pain receded I was able to jog a little faster. By the time I'd completed the 3.15 miles, the pain had subsided substantially. Two days later, when I jogged once more, the pain was much less, and it completely disappeared by the time I had completed my jog. By May 20 I had no sign of any back pain. Several months later I pulled a muscle in my leg. This time I decided to do nothing about the muscle or pain. No bandages, no wrapping, nothing. When I jogged the next time the pain was no different than when I had curried favor to the pain. In fact, the pain of the muscle disappeared just as rapidly as if I had favored it with wrapping and other care. Thereafter, I never curried favor to a torn muscle. The pain has always disappeared just as rapidly, if not more rapidly. This result really surprised me.

Beginning September 2, 1997, the next three jogs took almost thirty minutes for me to finish. On September 9, 1997, around my thirtieth anniversary of beginning to jog, I could not finish because of shortness of breath. I went home and called Dr. Siegel who asked me to come to his office. He determined that I had developed atrial fibrillation. Dr. Siegel prescribed Coumadin. This was the first time since I began jogging that I'd ever used medication for my heart condition. By September 21 the atrial fibrillation had disappeared and my jogging time remained between twenty-nine and thirty minutes. I stopped drinking coffee or consuming anything containing caffeine. Dr. Siegel authorized me to stop taking the coumadin six months later.

Referring back to the day I quit smoking, remember that my doctor told me I could develop gangrene in my feet if I continued to smoke? Well, about this time one of my barbers in Santa Clara who was in his sixties was being treated for gangrene in his feet and lower legs. His doctor told him that the gangrene was a result of his smoking. I asked the barber if he was now going to quit smoking to try to save his legs. His answer was that he would not quit because he liked smoking too much. He said he would rather lose his feet and legs than quit smoking. His doctor was trying to work out a schedule to amputate his feet up to the part of his legs where the gangrene had reached. The barber died before the operations were performed.

Dr. Jack Siegel has given me a semiannual medical exam since 1994. He gave me several treadmill tests up to 1997. In October 1997, he began the annual use of a treadmill stress test. He begins his treadmill with the floor raised to the first level of incline and a slow pace, then increases the incline and pace every three minutes. My test continued for nine and one-half minutes. During the next several years my time increased to ten minutes. Dr. Siegel's comparison chart showed my capacity to be higher than the average forty-five year old man.

By 1998, my jogging time was up to 31 minutes on average for the 3.15 miles. My weight was 160 pounds and my blood pressure was 110/70. My pulse rate was about 56. On February 17, 1998, I experienced atrial fibrillation again. I didn't tell anyone about it, and it went away within a couple of days. My heartbeat was irregular for a couple of days, and my time increased by two and one-half minutes for one jog of 3.15 miles. In 1998, I reduced the amount of weights I used for the bench press to 65 pounds on each arm with the repetitions at 18, 16, and 14. I changed one arm curl from 45 pounds to 35 pounds in each arm, and kept the push-ups and dips at the same level. My time remained between 29 and 32 minutes until December 10, 1998, when it went up to 33 minutes four times during the next three months. Then it dropped back to an average between 30 and 32 minutes.

In the winter of 1998, I was jogging along Blossom Hill Road between Walnut Blossom and Beswick when two fire trucks traveled east with their sirens blaring. I thought to myself that they were on the other side of the street and, at least, I'd have no reason to worry about those trucks interfering with my jog. Well, they pulled across the Beswick intersection turning north into the Magic Sands mobile home community, stopped in the pedestrian lane and blocked my path. How wrong I was. I lost a minute on my jogging time, but the fire trucks were gone the next time I was out. This is really a side issue, but it reminded me of the many times in my life that I have been wrong in my assumptions. In fact, I think that I've been wrong ninety-nine percent of the time when I've made assumptions. I'm really no good at guessing.

On April 13, 1999, I stopped writing down comments and just recorded the time of the jog. In reviewing the record from 1991 to April 10, 1999, I find that about one-third of the time I recorded having sore muscles. On April 10 I stopped recording how I felt during or after the jog, and most of those pains have deserted my memory. I remember the torn Achilles tendon while I was in Anderson, Indiana, and the last time I had back pain. I also remember the times I tumbled down the street and slid down the sidewalk, but most of the painful stress memories are gone. Isn't it funny that pain disappears from my mind unless I develop a method of keeping track of it? I only recorded pulling a back muscle using the weights and pulling a muscle under my right ribs after that date. I recorded those pains using an asterisk because they were unusually painful.

I no longer belong to a spa or YMCA, so I can't find a facility to use during my travels. As a result, when traveling I jog and do push-ups, but none of the other resistance exercises. My strength disappears quickly if I don't maintain the exercise on a regular schedule. Whenever I travel from San Jose to another state it takes me several weeks to get enough strength back to complete my weight lifting routine.

On August 28, 1999, I changed my jogging route, which increased the distance to 3.4 miles. This is the day I decided to jog at a pace that didn't strain any of my muscles. I go south to Blossom Hill Road, east to the Cottle-Hayes intersection, west on Hayes, and back home. I jog twice around the circuit from my house on Walnut Blossom Drive. My time also changed. It jumped up to 35'24" for the 3.4 miles, then back down to 33 minutes.

On November 9, 2000, I reached age seventy. My jogging and resistance exercising continued at pretty much the same pace. My routine didn't change; it was just a natural part of my life.

In 2001 Leslie and Jeff divorced. My jogging time stayed between 33 and 36 minutes until February 2002, when it moved up to over 36 minutes.

In 2001 I decided to complete my college education. (I had attended the University of Utah for one semester in 1953.) I'm now working on an Economics degree at San Jose State University. In February 2002 my astronomy professor at Evergreen Valley College, Mr. Michael M. Masuda, told the class that oxygen cleanses our blood stream and rejuvenates our bodies.[2] I'm convinced fresh oxygen is the greatest medicine available. This book is trying to convey that message to the readers.

---

2. I'm not aware of any controlled studies showing the effects of using oxygen versus not using oxygen. Consider a group of 5,000 people, one-half uses oxygen for twenty years and the other half uses no oxygen for twenty years. Which group would show the greatest benefit?

On March 21, 2002, my brother Leo passed away at age sixty-eight. Leo had remarkable determination and stamina. He lived quite a few years longer than even he thought he would live and many years longer than a person with less determination. He suffered from heart failure, emphysema, cancer, and other medical maladies. His funeral services were held in Salt Lake City. My brother Junius and I shared a motel room when we attended the services. The day before the service, I jogged for about forty-five minutes near the motel. When I returned, Junius told me that my face was as red as a beet. The jog was exhausting. The cause was a combination of tension arising from the funeral and the altitude at Salt Lake City. Two days later my jog was more normal and my face looked normal at the end even though I jogged a greater distance. I was seventy-one years old.

In 2002, my grandson Rob graduated from North Eugene High School in Eugene, Oregon, and entered Oregon State University at Corvallis. Angela graduated from Oak Grove High School in San Jose, California, and decided to work before continuing her education. Stacey entered Oak Grove High School and Rachel entered North Eugene High School. Wendy and Doug Sabin divorced. We're all getting older. The generations are taking their turns at the new stages of life.

In Mid-September 2002, I completed thirty-five years of jogging. My time stayed between 35 and 37 minutes for the 3.4 miles until October 12, 2002. On October 12 my time jumped up to 39'04". On October 15, 2002, I began my regular jog at a little after 6:15 AM. *At 6:25 AM, I had covered about 8/10 of a mile when suddenly my heart raced and it felt like it tried to stop beating. My heart acted and felt like a bird in the sky being knocked for a loop by a bullet, then fluttering its wings, trying to keep in the air.* I was passing a six foot high fence and grabbed onto the fence to keep from falling down. The pain was sudden and intense, I couldn't breathe and gasped for air. I had passed a couple of pedestrians who were walking west in the direction of Oak Grove High School and were now out of sight around the bend. I thought about calling out for help, but decided they wouldn't be able to hear me. Magic Sands mobile home community is on the other side of the fence and I thought if I called for help it would only frighten those living in the mobile homes. In any event, I thought help would come too late. As I gasped for air I considered lying down on the ground, but decided if I did lie down, I would lose consciousness and would lose all semblance of control. I decided to hold onto the fence and try to get air into my lungs and bring the beating of my heart under control. Within a minute or two I could start breathing again and my heart started to beat irregularly, but it was still beating. My ability to breathe as I had before the event was severely hampered. It is my belief that holding onto the fence and remaining upright kept me alive. I decided to continue on my jogging route. I walked a short distance, then jogged slowly for a little while. I completed the 3.4 mile distance, but I had to stop and walk three different times. At first I thought it was atrial fibrillation run amok. But then I concluded it was a heart attack because my heart would not allow the same degree of exertion. It was my reduced capacity and the increase in the length of time it took me to complete my jog that lead me to believe it was a heart attack. I did not check with my doctor at this time. My advice to anyone reading this book is to immediately check with your own doctor if this ever happens to you. I felt at the time that I needed to take this risk and it might have been quite foolish.

Two days after the event I began to walk around the jogging loop. I walked the 3.4 miles for a week, then tried jogging again. I jogged very slowly for about two weeks and continued to use the weights after my jog. I began to feel exhausted during the day of my jog, my breathing was not right and there was an inadequate oxygen supply to my lungs. I felt like I was breathing stale air and that my body was worn out and it just didn't respond like it used to. I decided to reduce my exercise routine. I started walking instead of jogging the full 3.4 miles. It took me about 54 minutes to walk the route. I got that down to 50 minutes in a week and 47 minutes in three weeks.

I also reduced my weights so that I only do 50 push-ups, used only the 25-pound weights for my arm exercises, which I increased to four sets of ten repetitions. I took 20 pounds off the weights for the bench press. The bench press weights were now at 55 pounds in each arm. I reduced the number of dips to 25 reps. This made a lot of difference in how I felt.

Around October 30 I had a dream where my deceased brother, David, and my deceased brother-in-law, Dan Collier, were in a limousine with Dan driving and David in the passenger seat. I called to them to let me in the back seat of the car, but they ignored me and started to drive off. I called again and ran to the car, opened the back door and tried to climb in, but there was a drop down table covering the back seat which left no room for me to sit. They continued to ignore me and drove off. The passenger door where David was sitting and the back passenger side door where I tried to climb into the car were both open as they drove away. My interpretation of this dream is that I was concerned about my own possible death, but my brother, David, would have none of it. He felt that I should continue living at this time.

In November 2002, my statistics professor at Evergreen Valley College, Robert Knight, MD, a medical doctor who tired of all insurance paperwork and decided to teach school, explained to the class that the first heart attack for men younger than age thirty-five will probably be fatal, while men over age fifty-five have a greater chance of surviving the first heart attack. The reason is that older men have developed more "feeder" arteries which can take over in the event a major artery is blocked. He said that currently one-third of all heart attack sufferers die with the first attack.

I visited with my cardiologist, Dr. Siegel, on January 14, 2003. I should have seen him on October 15, 2002, but there were personal reasons for the delay, not a death wish. He completed a stress test with an ECG on the treadmill and an echocardiogram. Dr. Siegel concluded I had had an episode of nonsustained ventricular tachycardia and a renewal of atrial fibrillation. I'd never heard of ventricular tachycardia, but it is where the heart beat can be initiated in the lower heart chamber rather than the upper heart chamber. The heart can beat between 140 and 230 beats a minute. Ventricular tachycardia requires immediate emergency care. Atrial fibrillation is where the atria, the upper chambers of the heart, can beat irregularly and very rapidly. It can beat somewhere between 300 to 500 bpm. As a result, the ventricle can beat at rates between 80 and 160 bpm. They are really out of sync and the doctor needs to bring them back into sync. It is common in atherosclerotic disease, which is my problem. My heartbeat on that day was 110. Dr. Siegel has prescribed coumadin and beta blockers. This is the second time that I've used medication for my heart disease. Dr. Siegel and I discussed completing an angiogram because of the rhythm disturbance and my reduced capacity over the last year.

On January 16, 2003, I walked 2.8 miles, then jogged for one hundred paces, walked and jogged five more times to the end of the 3.4 mile distance. My time was 46'23''. Again, I felt stale air in my lungs at the end of the jog. On January 18 I did the same thing, but I didn't feel stale air at the end. My time was 45'25''. It is my recollection that Dr. Siegel told me five or six years ago that after the first heart attack a person can expect another attack about ten years later. It has been about thirteen years since my last heart attack.

I met with Dr. Siegel again on January 21, 2003, and discussed this same issue with him. He said he doesn't remember the conversation, but that my interpretation isn't correct. He said the results of angioplasty will either fail within six months or will last for many years. He said cholesterol can build up around the stent, but not at any faster rate than in the other arteries. He said it is true that the blockage of one artery can mean there will be other arteries blocked in the future, but the rate of incidence rests with the lifestyle of the patient. In my case, my exam still shows a strong heart. Dr. Siegel said that with proper medication, I should be able to get back to my regular jogging routine.

My heartbeat reached 199 on the treadmill. My blood pressure was 110/72, and my resting heartbeat after ingesting coumadin and the beta blockers is 60. On January 21, 2003, Dr. Siegel said that I should have another ten years to live. He said that his major concern at this time is stroke. He said atrial fibrillation contributes to strokes on a compounding basis. He said that under these conditions strokes can be postponed, but not totally eliminated.

On January 21st I walked and then jogged 150 paces, 4 times during the last half mile. I felt okay. My time was 45'05''. On January 23rd, I walked and jogged the last mile very slowly. My time was 45'08''. I felt okay and experienced no stale air. On January 25th, I jogged and walked intermittently. I jogged for about a quarter mile, then walked for about an eighth of a mile. I continued the same pattern for the 3.4 miles. My time was 39´46˝. I was tired at the end, but had no feeling of stale air. (The advice I get from those close to me is to slow down, do less. They're afraid the strain on my heart will be fatal. I don't think so.)

On January 30, 2003, my jog and walk time was forty minutes even. I met with Dr. Siegel again. He said that my blood pressure was 110/70, but the rate of my heartbeat was 117 bpm. He said that he wanted to do a cardioversion (defibrillator) procedure, which is an electric shock treatment, on February 13th and an angiogram on February 20th. I agreed to both procedures and they were scheduled. The rapid heartbeat caused my body to warm up much more than normal. The room felt much warmer than usual when I went to bed at night l. I'd get so warm that I'd have to remove a couple of blankets in order to sleep. Usually when I sleep, I get cold and need an extra blanket later at night or towards morning. My usual pulse rate would drop down to between 50 and 60 beats per minute during rest at night. At over 100 bpm, the blood rushing through the body creates heat that I usually only experience when exercising.

Dr. Siegel also prescribed flecainide medication. Flecainide has a side effect of causing constipation and blurred vision. When I began to jog my stomach felt as though I had just eaten a complete meal. It was difficult to overcome the heaviness in my stomach and jog naturally. As a result, I ate prunes and more fruit.

On February 13, 2003, Dr. Siegel performed cardioversion. I asked the anesthesiologist why anesthesia was necessary if the shock only lasted one or two seconds. He told me that it is very painful. I asked Dr. Siegel the same question, and he said that one of his professors in medical school had the same question so he tied the gadget to his leg and gave himself one-fourth of the normal shock. The professor said it felt like he had placed his leg in a bucket of molten lava. Dr. Siegel also said that even when a person is in dire straights and the application of Cardioversion is necessary, they are supposed to wait until the person is unconscious before performing the procedure because of the pain. My cardioversion required two shocks instead of just one. I was under the anesthetic for about five minutes and when I awoke I could feel tingling in the ends of my nerves on my legs, arms, and chest. So I guess the doctors were right. One residual effect of the shock treatment was a feeling of soreness in the right side of my jaw. The second day after the treatment, as I went outside to jog, my right ear had pain. Later in the day when I began to eat breakfast, the right side of my jaw felt the same pain as I bit down on food. The right side of my jaw had pain for about five days after the cardioversion. I was probably biting down on my jaw when the shock was applied.

On February 20, 2003, I jogged for the entire 3.4 miles, even though it was a very slow jog. Jogging is harder than walking, even at the same time and distance. A person lifts his body off the ground with each jog step, but remains on the ground when walking. On this same day Dr. Siegel completed the angiogram. He found no significant blockage or cholesterol problems which would require performing angioplasty. He said that even though there is some cholesterol buildup it isn't significant enough to worry about. I guess clean living has paid off. So, the major thrust for me from here on out will be to control the atrial fibrillation. Har, har, har, har, staying alive, staying alive.

On April 15, 2003, Dr. Siegel completed another treadmill stress test and found most of my capacity had returned, my test was still better than a healthy forty-five year old male. There was no ischemia, no arrhythmia, the heart rate was low, under sixty beats a minute, and my blood pressure was 115/70. He said he would probably keep me on Coumadin for another six months. I told him that my legs feel heavy while jogging, and I have a loss of muscle strength. He said this might be caused by the medication, but there might be some other source, so he'll continue the current medication and later see if there is some method of comparing results to find the cause of the loss of muscle strength.

My weight moved up to between 163 and 165 pounds during this uncertain period. By April 29, 2003, I was up to 165. So I began to drink orange juice (which is normal) after my jog and then just eat the grapefruit for breakfast. I postponed eating my Raisin Bran and Fiber One until noon on the days I jogged. By June 7, my weight was back down to 160.

On May 13, 2003, I met with Dr. Siegel and he advised me that there is a possibility in the future of installing a pacemaker. I asked him how it would affect my jogging, and he said it would not make any difference. He said that the new pacemakers adjust to the needs of the heart, but control the beats so the rhythm is in line with medical requirements. We also reviewed my medication. I told him that the beta blockers seem to make my legs harder to move in the jog. He agreed that it could happen, and we discussed reducing the amount of dosage. Dr. Siegel advised me to reduce the dosage by one-half. My beta blocker, Toprol XL, dose was 100 mg once a day. That was reduced to 50 mg. I also take 120 mg Armour thyroid (which I've taken since age twenty-five), 50 mg Flecainide, 5 mg warfarin (Coumadin), and 81 mg aspirin. I take a multiple vitamin tablet, folic acid, and 65 mg iron tablet.

On June 10, 2003, Dr. Siegel suggested that I stay on the same medication for the next two months. He also said that there is research on atrial fibrillation that seems to imply that in five years there will be a procedure to eliminate it.

On June 12, 2003, I developed a serious pain on the left side of my left foot. It was in the tendon area just above my arch. I hoped to work out the pain by just leaving it alone, but when it became worse I decided to see Dr. Meltzer. On June 19, Dr. Meltzer x-rayed my foot to see if the bone had splintered. It had not. I had pulled a tendon, so he gave me a cortisone shot. My jog on June 21 created a serious shortness of breath. I couldn't finish the six tenths mile warmup jog. I then jogged much slower during the regular 3.4 mile jog. The first two miles were hard, but my breathing began to get better during the last part of the jog. Cortisone might have caused some of the effect, but I really don't know whether it was the cortisone or temporary atrial fibrillation. My jogging time now runs from 39 to 42 minutes. It stays around 40 minutes most of the time, but will increase when I'm facing a stressful situation. My time reduces when everything seems pleasant and relaxing.

On July 1, 2003, I increased the amount of weights I use for the bench press.

In November 2003 I reached seventy-three years of age. In December I reduced the Toprol to 12.5 mg and jogged. The first jog felt pretty good and my time was a little under 40 minutes for the 3.4 miles. But on the fourth jogging day I felt atrial fibrillation at the end of the jog. I had to stop jogging and walk. So, I increased the Toprol back to 50 mg. Obviously, my heart will need constant monitoring for the balance of my life.

On December 31, 2003, I increased the number of repetitions on the bench press.

In March 2004, my new general practitioner decided to put me on Zocor in addition to my other heart medication. I tried it for a few days but the reaction on my body was quite severe. It gave me muscle aches, diarrhea, sweats, and chills. I stopped the Zocor, but the adverse effects remained for several more weeks.

On August 26, 2004, I was doing bench presses when a spider crawled up my nose. I tried to blow it out, but it just kept climbing up higher. I put down the weights and blew and wiped the spider out. Then I decided to start over on my bench presses. I pressed too many repetitions and pulled the muscles on the left side of my ribs. It took about a month for the ribs to heal. Then in October, I got a flu shot. The needle was pushed into a muscle and caused my muscle to hurt when I used the weights. It's now the end of the year and my arm muscle is just now beginning to feel better.

I'm taking several courses at San Jose State University and Evergreen Valley College. I had difficulty concentrating on the Calculus problems so I decided to see what happened when I reduced the distance of my jog and changed the days of my jog. I jogged on the days that I did not attend classes. I found that by reducing the distance to 2.2 miles from 3.4 miles it did not make me quite as tired and my concentration improved. So, my actual jogging distance is .6 mile as a warm-up and 2.2 miles for the regular jog.

In October 2004 I developed problems with my hemorrhoids. I didn't want to have an operation during my school year, so I waited until Christmas before scheduling an operation. On January 7, 2005, Dr. Mark M. Segall performed the operation. He's an excellent surgeon. On January 10th I was back at my normal routine, except I lowered the amount of weights on my bench press for two weeks. I jogged the 2.2 (plus .6) miles at a slower pace. The next jog was my normal time, and by January 17th my time was down to 27 ′30 ″.

My wife, Dorothy, began walking on a regular schedule towards the end of 2003. Her diabetes was having a negative effect on her. She was exhausted and couldn't walk 100 yards. She decided to do her best to increase her walking distance and would walk an extra ten or fifteen paces each day. Soon, she was walking a quarter mile. Then she was able to walk a half mile. Then, after several months, she was walking almost a mile. Now she walks about one and one quarter miles four or five times a week. Her health has improved dramatically. She's much more active and does much more housework as well as shopping. Her diabetes medication has been reduced dramatically. She's only one month younger than I am.

The years are many. I'm past my thirty-seventh year at this writing. My experiences are varied, and the knowledge I have is that which can only be gained through experience. My wife and I have had as many serious family and business problems as any other marriage will suffer. There've been good times and bad. There's been muscle pain and feelings of well-being that can't be duplicated in any other way. Through it all, I'm still alive. My decision was to take control of my body and I think I've done that.

Part II
My Family

The health and exercise routine of my immediate family members as well as brothers and sisters needs to be inserted in this book. Some readers might wonder how my family has responded to my life experiences based upon the changes to my health and body. They will tell you in their own words a little bit about their health and their routines.

My wife, Dorothy, has done some exercising. She continued to live in Salt Lake City from 1980 to 1986, and for several years she would take brisk walks along the roads in her neighborhood. She decided that walking would be a good form of exercise for her. Then she stopped exercising for the next seventeen years. In 2003 walking seemed to be hard for her and she didn't find it very interesting. Her energy was depleted and she really didn't feel like getting out of her chair in the living room. She did start walking again in early 2003. It was very hard for her at first, but she gradually built her distance up to about one and one-quarter miles. Then she stopped again. But in 2004 she started walking again and her health is much improved. Her energy is coming back and she's feeling much better.

My brother, Leo, who was almost three years younger than I, never engaged in a sustained exercise program. He wrote this unsolicited e-mail message to me and my brothers, Harold, Conrad, and Junius, on February 20, 2000:

I was fussing around the apartment a week or so ago, and I came across my copies of the hospital records which I needed when I submitted for Long term Disability in 1994. I had, often, wondered where these were, but never did a serious search for them; and, lo and behold when I was looking for something else, these jumped out and said, "Grab me!" So, I did.

Tonight, the mood struck me to solve a trivia curiosity of long standing. I sat down and counted the number of times I had been in the hospital to deal with my bladder cancer harvestings. Since January, was the fourteenth year anniversary of dealing with this unpublished story, and my doctor developooed (sic) a parallel empathy about my extractions to inform me, this last visit at LDS Hospital, I, finally, had the mood strick (sic) me to count the total visits.

My current Urologist, Dr. Chidester, let me know that the computer record showed that my most recent visit and operation was the fourteenth time since 1993. My records gave me a count of thirteen operations prior to that. So, the total operations have been 27, to date.

All of these hospital visits do not include the number Cystoscope examination, which have been every 3 months since the beginning. That makes 56 of those. And, then we have to include Thiotepa and BCG treatments, which meant six weeks of each series: Thiotepa, being 6 weeks; BCG being 20 treatments (one series stopped after the first or second application); and, then one Adriamiacin treatment: these are all concidered (sic) as chemotherapy.

Add all of these invasions to my bladder, we get a grand total of 96 (+ or –).

This is not to be bragging, or anything of that nature, because I think that Harold and Kurt have survived health risks much more serious than mine; and, I applaud them for their success and great attitudes after all is said and done.

Please, remember, this is just one of those weird "Trivia" curiousity (sic) attacks.

So, Have fun, and be good to each other.

As Always,
Leoj.
Pogo sez; "We have met the enemy, and they is Us."

(Kurt Jensen is a cousin who nearly died as a result of Type I diabetes and had several organ transplants that allowed him to live. He has written his own story and it's worth reading.)

My oldest brother, Harold, and I worked together in the life insurance company in Salem, Oregon, from the fall in 1959 to the spring in 1969. In 1968 Harold began jogging. He could see the improvement on my body and decided to do the same for himself. On January 28, 2002, Harold sent this message to me after I asked him for comments to include in this book:

I don't recall the month I started jogging, but it was in the summer or early fall of 1968. The first triple bypass was in June 1974. On December 7, 1973, I had some chest pains and was barely able to feed the animals we had at that time. So, I went in to see Harmon (Dr. Harmon T. Harvey). He thought it was probably not a heart attack, but he sent me to the hospital to have them take a blood sample. They found enzymes in the blood that are the result of a heart episode. Harmon then said I had a heart attack, Apparently it was not the result of a thrombus, but rather a severe restriction of the three coronary arteries. He sent me home to stay in bed for a while, then In June of 1974 he sent me up to Dr. U. Scott Page, who was with Northwest Surgical Associates in Portland. He and Dr. Bigelow did an angiogram and advised me that it was either immediate heart surgery or die. They scheduled me right in. Then 19 years later, in August of 1993, the arteries had plugged up again. The angiogram indicated a similar problem and the second triple bypass was performed. It was interesting: in the first surgery Dr. Page was the lead surgeon and Dr. Bigelow assisted; in the second one the roles were reversed. Dr. Page assisted Dr. Bigelow. The first surgery was done at Good Samaritan Hospital in Portland. The second was done in Salem's Memorial Hospital. The doctors felt that 19 years on the first bypasses was an excellent record, the average being 10 years.

I have gone for 9 years on the second one and am not a candidate for a third heart surgery. I am being treated with medications and doing relatively well. It is quite remarkable. It has been 28 years since the first bypass surgery. That means I have lived more than one-third of my life since the first surgery. I am quite convinced I could not have lived these last 27 years if I had not been jogging as a result of your persuasion. Thanks.

Hank.

Harold amended his message to me so that I could include the length of time he has continued his exercising. That amendment follows:

Hi Reg:

When I started walking in Pacific Palisades (California) in 1968, I could hardly make it around the block. By the time we got home (Salem, Oregon) in 1969, I could barely walk down the hill to the mailbox from our home and had to walk back up in stages. Eventually I was able to walk down and back. Then started jogging a little bit at a time. In a year or so, I was jogging about 2.5 miles every other day in the not very fast time of 35 minutes. I kept this up for about 27 years, then gradually began to slow down for want of stamina. About seven years ago I was no longer able to jog and settled for walking about the same distance. Then gradually the distances got shorter. After the pacemaker was installed, about 5 years ago, my heart began relying on the pacemaker 100 percent of the time. It was set at 70 beats per minute. This limited my walking more. Now I walk with a cane about one-half mile irregularly as I feel up to it.

I have survived about 30 years from the first heart attack and open-heart surgery and 11 years from the second. During this later period, I had gal (sic) bladder surgery and colon cancer surgery with a colostomy and have survived that, so far, for 5 years. There is no doubt in my mind that if I had not started the aerobic exercise you recommended, after reading Dr. Kenneth H. Cooper's book, "Aerobics," I would have been dead by age 50. Of course, I have had extremely good medical care along the way. In combination, they have given me 30 years of extra good life.

Hank."

Harold, had been jogging for five years when he had his heart attack. His doctor told him that his exercise routine contributed to saving his life.

On January 30, 2002, my next eldest brother, Lt. Col. (Ret) Hyrum Conrad Jensen had this to say about his heart problems (he was age fifty-four in 1980):

Dear Reg:

I had a mild heart attack in about 1980. I had an angiogram performed. There was minor blockage in one small vessel of the heart. I was informed the body would develop new channels to feed that part of the heart. I have been on various medications since. And I have been under cardiologist care since.

I did not have angina. I did not have angioplasty. I was shown the film of the angiogram it showed blockage at the extreme end of one small artery which stopped blood flow to that small portion of the heart muscle. But it was minor and my cardiologist who did the angiogram said the body would develop a new route to feed that portion (because it was minor).

I have had various kinds of stress tests over the years and one additional angiogram last year. My blockage is still minor.

Hope this helps. Good luck on the book.

Conrad, at age seventy-six, found that his breathing is restricted, so he's taken up walking. He now walks about one and one-quarter miles and expects to get the distance up to two miles. He visited with Dorothy and me in the summer of 2003 and walked around my jogging circuit (1.7 miles) every day. He said that walking in San Jose is much easier than it is in Florida. It would be so because of the Florida humidity.

Our eldest daughter, Wendy, keeps her weight down and keeps active with her children and work, but she's never instituted a regular exercise routine. She once told me that she went for a five mile walk with her friends and her body ached for several days after that.

Wed, 8 Jan 2003 19:50:35-0800

Dad,

Unfortunately I don't do any regular exercise routine with the exception of the following: I do sit ups (sic) almost every morning as soon as I get up and while I'm waiting for my coffee water to heat. Then I ride my bicycle with Sage every morning for 15–30 minutes. Before last January, I did two bicycle rides with her every day. This probably isn't great exercise for me since I have to go a pace that works for Sage's shorter legs. I keep her going at somewhat of a pace and sometimes she breaks loose and runs but it still doesn't tax me at all. In the past I have done lots of exercise things like taking jazzersie (sic) classes etc, but that was when the kids were very small or before they were born. I've taken water aerobics once too. Last year I did Tai chi for 9 months. I'd like to get into a regular routine with yoga and Tai chi again but it doesn't count until I do! I'm starting a walking routine with Sage now—in addition to the bicycle every morning, I'm taking her for a fast (fast for me) walk in the evenings 3–4 days a week. I'm starting with about 4 blocks and will increase this as the days get longer and I have more light to walk. I have done lot's (sic) of hiking in the past but again it was long ago..oh just remembered that I did do a regular 30 minute workout on the Nordic track for about 6 months several years ago but haven't recently.

Hope this info helps!

Love Wendy

I asked our middle daughter, Cindy to give me her history of exercising. Here is what she wrote.

Date: Fri, 3 Jan 2003 17:21:13-0800

To: Dad

OK—let's see 1956–1968: From birth to 6th grade I don't remember much of anything regarding exercise other than regular playground play and regular youngster play. There was nothing organized and I was not a member of any sporting activity.

1968–1971: In 7th–9th grade I participated in P.E. class in school, but did not do any other sports or regular exercise. In the summer 8th grade, I began swimming at nights in the summer. I swam hard and for a few hours. During that summer I lost a lot of weight. I became a "regular" sized girl as opposed to an overweight girl. 1971–1974: In high school I did not participate in any sports and do not remember exercising.

1974–1978: In college I began riding my bicycle a lot and walking a lot to classes. My classes were about 1–2 miles from the dorm, so I walked or rode my bicycle everyday to and from class. In college I participated in a synchronized swimming class and club. I also participated in some dancing classes. In college I also took a belly dancing class. I do not remember doing any regular exercise in college other than bicycling, walking, swimming and belly dancing. 1978–1980: In graduate school I began jogging a little. I do not remember how regular I was with this exercise. I also joined gyms and worked out at gyms sometimes.

1980–82: When I moved to New Jersey, I began jogging more regularly and working out on the Nautilus equipment (weight training). I was in the best shape at that time. I also swam. I jogged 3–5 miles approximately 3 times/week (I think) and I worked out with the Nautilus three times/week. I was consistent with that for about two years. I also played racquetball. I played racquetball about once per week. 1982–1986: In Virginia, I began exercising at the gym in aerobics classes and working out on the exercise equipment. I also ran. I would swim 1 mile a few times/week. I consistently exercised while in Virginia for about one year. I then bought a Nordic Track machine and began cross country skiing. I also did aerobics tapes. I sometimes jogged. I was fairly consistent with this exercise, but I began gaining weight in Virginia and DC.

1986–1990: During this time I was sporadic with exercise but dabbled in it. Sometimes I would get motivated and do a lot of aerobics tapes. Sometimes I would be jogging. Sometimes I would do the Nordic Track. I took golf lessons at this time. 1990–1998: During this time the most exercise I got was cleaning houses. I also began walking during this time. I got a LOT of exercise cleaning houses.

1998–PRESENT: I did not exercise very much when I first started the police department. However, during the past year I have been better at exercising. I either do aerobics tapes, the treadmill, walking, or the Nordic Track. I was doing this exercise 4–5 times per week for about 7–8 months. Then I lost the motivation. I am now doing Cardio Kickboxing 4–5 times per week for 45 minutes.

Here I thought I was a good exerciser, but I realize when I put it in writing that I have been very inconsistent and not so good. I see that I would be good for a year or two at a time and then fall off for a year or two. I have always THOUGHT about exercising and have gotten back to it, but I haven't stayed on any one particular program like you have consistently for years.

Cindy has acted as a team leader for several Walks for Diabetes. She organized a group of walkers, then urged them to raise money for the Diabetes Foundation. She's been very successful in her efforts.

Our youngest daughter, Leslie, did try jogging and other exercises for about a year around 1993. Here are her comments:

This is my experience with "exercise." Precisely "jogging."

My dad told me that if I began to jog, that I would feel healthier. He has been the most health conscious person I have ever known. He had completely turned his life around, from what used to be a self-destructive one, to a life of someone who really wanted to live. I quite admire him, as does everyone who knows him. He is the ultimate role model. So, I decided to try his advice.

I remember the first time I went out with him for our two-mile run. I ended up half walking, half jogging. I barely made it home. I was panting, sweating, sore, and felt like my face and body was near on fire from heat and exertion.

Nevertheless, that did not discourage me from going out again, and again. We went every other day, early in the morning. I am not a morning person. Never have been. I prefer to be left alone then, because I am grouchy to have to get up out of bed early. But after the run, my mood would be completely different. I was elated and proud. Obviously, I was feeling physically good.

The runs got easier with a little time. Sometimes I would run in the evening instead, due to my schedule. Either way worked out well. Soon, my jogging turned into almost sprinting. I put the walkman (sic) on, and as I listened to my favorite music, the difficulty of this exercising, vanished away. I honestly then looked very forward to my jogging. Getting out there on the streets was peaceful, by myself, to run my stresses free. I felt good. I lost weight. I became stronger, physically.

I felt my lungs pump air, my heart beat well, the toxins spill out of my pores, my legs build strength and shape, and all my senses come more alive. At the end of my two miles, approaching home again, I sometimes felt like I could've just kept going and run another couple of miles, easy. That is when I felt my best.

I remember once that I pulled my sciatic nerve in my back. Normally I would've assumed that I would now have to lay down flat on my back until the pain eased up. I felt like I couldn't move. My dad gave me his advise from his own experience, and said "just go ahead and run" anyway. I thought he was nuts at first. Then I thought, "well, what have I got to lose?" So, I forced myself up, and took off jogging. Sure enough, to my amazement, the pain almost immediately ceased. At the end of the run, there was no more pain. I would have never imagined that.

My dad has stayed alive and healthy. Based upon the heart disease, which runs in the family, he is 100% certain he wouldn't have live (sic) much past thirty or forty years old, had he not exercised faithfully. I am so very proud of him. I have been so lucky and happy to have my father alive and with us each day. What a gift he is! How better can someone show their love to their family, by making sure that they do all they can, to stay alive for them?

No one can compare, to my dad. ♥

Leslie Jensen Morrison (his daughter)

My youngest brother, Junius, has not maintained a regular exercise routine since leaving high school. He does walk the dogs and do yard work, but not a sustained exercise pace. None of my sisters have developed a regular exercise routine. In my family, participating in sports in high school seemed to set the tone for the gender gap in regards to exercising.

However, my younger sister, Jewel Berg, just found out (May 2005) that she has breast cancer. She'll need radiation and chemotherapy. She's very positive about her outcome. She's convinced the cancer will be placed into remission. She joined a health club several months back. She needs to have her knees replaced, so she can't walk for any distance. However, she does use the various types of equipment in the club and she'll continue to do so because she knows that exercise is one thing she can do to help herself while the doctors do their job.

Part III
What Have the Pros Found Out

With this brief chronology of events over the last thirty-seven years, I can now offer advice on how a person can control his or her body. First, I want to cite a few publications discussing health and heart issues. How strong are our bodies, how tenacious are our organs? We can find out for ourselves!

Heart attacks are different. The recurrence of a heart attack is different. Nineteen years passed before Harold had his second attack. It's been over twenty-two years since Conrad had his heart attack. It was about thirty years between Louis's heart attacks. He had his first heart attack in the mid-1960s. Leo never had a second heart attack, but his death was attributed to heart failure, among other causes. Mine were about three months apart. Part of the heart muscle dies with each occurrence, so there is a finite number we can survive prior to death.

Let's start with some of the problems that need to be overcome after a person begins an exercise program. If someone's young and heavy, that person must begin controlling body weight. I'm sure most young people don't have a death wish. I didn't when I was heavy. People just don't believe the excess weight is life threatening. One reason for this belief is that we look around and see so many other people who are overweight and they aren't dead. We don't go around the country and examine dead people. When we die we disappear from view. It's easy for us to believe heavy people live forever. So, we need to consider what others have discovered. An article in the *San Jose Mercury News,* by reporter Tanner,[1] competently

---

1. Tanner, Lindsey. "Study: Obese young men can lose decades of life" <u>The Mercury News</u>, 8 Jan. 2003, 6A.

discussed the issue of excess weight. "Being obese at age 20 can cut up to 20 years off a person's life, with the biggest impact on black men, according to yet another study that underscores the long-term dangers of being overweight." The study appeared in the *Journal of The American Medical Association*[2] and was led by University of Alabama Birmingham biostatistician David Allison. The article reported that obesity increases the risk for several life-threatening conditions, including heart disease, diabetes, and some kinds of cancer. In my business, I've continually told people that a dead man can't sign his name. Here, I'll say that a dead man can't change his mind and elect to change his habits if he's given another chance. Studies following people who gain weight in mid-life show they still reduce their life span by years.

Another article in the *San Jose Mercury News* by reporter Caruso[3], that appeared one day earlier says that people over age forty who are overweight are likely to die at least three years sooner than those who are thinner. Caruso obtained his information from a study that was conducted by Dutch researchers and was published in the January 7, 2003, issue of the *Annals of Internal Medicine.* To quote from the article "For smokers, the results were even worse. Obese female smokers lost 7.2 years compared with normal-weight non-smoking women. Obese male smokers lost 6.7 years compared with trim smokers, and 13.7 years compared with normal-weight non-smokers." The results were culled from statistics collected from 3,457 volunteers in Framingham, Massachusetts, from 1948 to 1990.

One purpose of this book is to demonstrate how to avoid premature death from heart attacks. I'm just one person, not an amalgamation of a massive study, but I'm convinced many people can achieve the same results I've achieved. The American Heart Association[4] says that there are 1,200,000 heart attacks each year in the United States and that roughly

---

2.   Fontaine, Kevin, MD, et.al. "Years of Life Lost Due to Obesity." Journal of the American Medical Association. 8 Jan 2003: Vol. 289, 187-193.
3.   Caruso, David B. "Overweight adults die 3 years sooner, study finds." The Mercury News. 7 Jan 2003, 7A.
4.   American Heart Association: http://www.americanheart.org/presenter. jhtml?identifier=4591. 21 June 2005.

494,000 Americans die from heart disease each year. Other studies say there are 1.5 million heart attacks each year. *The New York Times Almanac 1999*[5] says "Some 1.5 million people suffer heart attacks annually. One-third of those people do not survive. Of the survivors, 44 percent of the women and 27 percent of the men will die within one year." There are about 1.5 million people in Santa Clara County (Silicon Valley). Would it make an impact on us if everyone in Santa Clara County had a heart attack and one-third of them died all in one year?

Television station KPIX Channel 5 San Francisco, on January 14, 2003, carried a program on heart disease sponsored by Sutter Health. It was hosted by Ms. Kim Enstom and featured Drs. Diane Sobkowitz, Mark Waxman, Ulbrite Sujansky, Richard Gray, Coyness Aeneas, Jr., Jane Lambert, David Anderson, and Michael Ingham, as panelists. (I'm not able to footnote the credits.) The program included film clips featuring other doctors. These medical professionals claimed that 75% of heart attacks can be eliminated, that metabolic disease is inherited and begins at inception, and arteries fissure and crack with cholesterol. They said stress increases adrenaline and constricts arteries and stress is controllable. They also said that folic acid and vitamin B_6 are both helpful. The doctors affirmed heart disease is the number one killer of women, two times greater than cancer. This means to me that women need to pay attention to their hearts and physical condition. The major publicity surrounds breast cancer, yet breast cancer is only one of many different cancers, and all cancers in women are less fatal than heart attacks. With their survival rate so much lower during the first year after a heart attack it means to me that women pay the price for avoiding participating in sports and exercise programs.

Studies on women have dealt with factors other than exercise. I've written about eating right, exercise, and getting plenty of rest. Apparently, too much rest is just as bad for women as too little. *SBC Yahoo News*[6] ran a Reuters story in 2003 saying "Women who don't get enough sleep and

5. Wright, John G., ed. 1999 The New York Times Almanac, New York: Penquin, 1999.

6. Study Links Sleep Imbalance to Heart Attacks. Yahoo! News. Http:// www.yahoo.com 27 Jan. 2003.

those who sleep too much may both run a greater risk of getting heart disease than those who log eight hours a day." This conclusion was from a study of 121,700 female nurses that began in 1976. The risk for heart disease went up on both sides of the eight hours of sleep spectrum.

Atrial fibrillation is more dangerous in women than men. More men suffer from atrial fibrillation, but a study reported by Megan Rauscher inVascularWeb[7] showed that women who have atrial fibrillation are four times more likely to have a stroke than were men with the same disorder. Atrial fibrillation is the most common kind of heart rhythm abnormality. I'll write a little more about atrial fibrillation in a few pages.

Here's a story about a women whose accomplishments are outstanding. Reporter Mike Cassidy interviewed Catra Corbett in Fremont, California.[8] Corbett was thirty-six years old at that time and planned to run two marathons in one day. Ms. Corbett was quoted as saying "I was hanging out in nightclubs, drinking, partying,…getting into drugs, and doing speed." Then, she said she didn't want to live that way anymore, she wanted to feel good, to be healthy. So, she started exercising, started walking, then jogging, then ran a 10K and then was inspired to enter the San Francisco marathon. Several years later she was running 50 and 100 mile races. I would guess her heart was not damaged by her previous lifestyle.

Women might have a fear of being attacked by a man while jogging. The risk of attack is negated if you jog in a neighborhood during normal waking hours. Once you become a fixture, people will be watching for you and unwittingly become your guardians. It would be nice for a city to pave jogging tracks in neighborhood parks. The police could patrol the area, especially in the early morning or evening, to provide security for women.

For a woman, what do you think her physical condition would be like after five years of a program consisting of twenty minutes of cardiovascular exercise and twenty minutes of resistance exercise three times each week?

7.   Rauscher, Megan. <u>VascularWeb</u>.
     Http://svs.vascularweb.org/_CONTRIBUTION_PAGES/Medical_News_reuters/
     Atrial_Fibrillation_Conf…21 June 2005. Am J. Cardiol 2004;94:889-894.
8.   Cassidy. Mike. "Runner Seeing Double." <u>San Jose Mercury News</u>. 22 Oct. 2001:
     B1+.

She'd have her diet under control, her complexion under control, her physique under control. She'd probably survive any heart attack and escape most cancers. She'd also have her pick of partners.

How about the men? The *Journal of the American Medical Association* published an article entitled "Exercise Type and Intensity in Relation to Coronary Heart Disease in Men."[9] In discussing coronary heart disease, the article said: "A cohort of 44,452 United States men enrolled in the Health Professional's Follow-up Study, followed at two year intervals from 1986 through January 31, 1998, to assess potential CHD risk factors, identify newly diagnosed cases of CHD, and assess levels of leisure-time physical activity." The study found, with a 95% confidence level, adjusted for various factors, such as smoking, age, and other cardiovascular risks, that running for one hour or more per week had a 42% reduction in risk factors, weight training for thirty minutes or more per week had a 23% risk reduction, and rowing for one hour or more per week had a 18% risk reduction. The comparisons were with inactive men.

I think there have been enough studies which show smoking increases the risk of heart disease and cancer. Among my family, my siblings, and in-laws, there have been three incidents of emphysema and five incidents of cancer. Some of our partners have diabetes. Why should we use obesity, nicotine, or any other substance to assist us on the road to suicide? I believe we start out doing something we consider to be exciting. For the last several thousand years, drugs have been used to help people escape drudgery and tolerate boredom. Drudgery is spending months on a ship, building railroad tracks, being a slave laborer, and performing other demeaning tasks. The misuse of food and drugs is not exciting in the long run. A person should go ahead and do it, if necessary, get it out of the system, and get on with living. If you're going to live a dangerous lifestyle, no one can stop you, but you'll find it's a waste of time. Making a living can be pretty exciting at times without drugs, especially if a person's not able to meet the bills. Eating too much? The food tastes good, so it's easy to put

9.   Tanasescu, M. et.al. "Exercise Type and Intensity in Rrelation to Coronaray Heart Disease in Men." The Journal of the American Medical Association 23-30 Oct. 2002, 288(16) 419-20.

more in the mouth, which causes the stomachs to stretch, and the expanded stomach demands more food to fill it up.

In a front page article in the *San Jose Mercury News* in 2002, entitled "Survival of the Fittest,"[10] the article stated that "physical activity [has been] shown to be [the] best longevity gauge." The article goes on to say "If you want to do the most important thing you can to live a long life, buy a pair of athletic shoes—and use them. Personal fitness levels turned out to be the greatest predictor of how long someone might live—more important than smoking habits, having high blood pressure or a personal history of heart attacks—in a new study of more than 6,000 California men published in the New England Journal of Medicine." The study was carried out by Stanford University and the Veterans Affairs Palo Alto Health Care System and it was limited to men.

Quoting from another article discussing depression in the *Readers Digest*,[11] "Exercise for the Mind," "Reviewing 14 studies in which supervised exercise programs were used to treat clinical depression, researchers found that patients with mild to moderate depression who walked, ran or performed strength training three times a week for 20 to 60 minutes were significantly less depressed after as few as five weeks. Studies that tracked subjects for up to one year found that when workouts were kept up, the improvements continued. How physical activity keeps the mind fit isn't clear, but researchers speculate it may alter brain chemistry." In my opinion, it's the fresh oxygen passing through the blood stream that keeps the mind fit.

The study of heart disease continues and more new facts are uncovered. For example, an article by Daniel Haney titled "Hidden factor in Heart Disease,"[12] says research finds inflammation triggers heart attacks. "New research suggests that inflammation, as measured by C-reactive protein (CRP), is an even more important trigger." Someone with the highest

10.   Lyons, Julie Sevrens. "Survival of the Fittest." The San Jose Mercury News." 14 Mar. 2002, final ed., A1+.
11.   Psychology Today. "Exercise for the Mind." Readers Digest Mar. 2002: 44.
12.   Haney, Daniel Q. "Hidden Factor in Heart Disease." *San Jose Mercury News.* August 4, 2002: A16.

combination of cholesterol and C-reactive protein has 8.7 times the risk of heart attack as someone with the lowest combination. The article lists those conditions which put you at risk: increasing age, being male, having parents with heart disease, smoking, total cholesterol over 239, HDL, the "good" cholesterol, below 35, high blood pressure, lack of physical activity, being overweight, and diabetes. All of the studies continue to show the same results, a regular exercise program is vital in sustaining a healthy body.

The *San Jose Mercury News* periodically runs profiles of different people and their exercise routine under the title "How I Stay Fit." Most of the people featured in these articles are joggers and most of them are between the ages of forty and sixty. I believe the articles are published once a week.

Reporter Steve Sternberg[13] writes:

The studies, focusing on different populations totaling about half a million people, indicate that about 90% of people with severe heart disease have one or more of four classic risk factors: smoking, diabetes, high cholesterol and high blood pressure.

That means the vast majority of the 650,000 new heart attacks each year could be prevented or delayed for decades by quitting smoking, reducing cholesterol and controlling hypertension and diabetes.

"If we could eliminate smoking and get people to be fit and trim, we could turn this thing around without unraveling the genes that cause heart disease," says researcher Eric Topol of the Cleveland Clinic Foundation. He is co-author of a study involving more than 120,000 heart patients.

I made some notes on an article quoting Dr. Philip Greenland of Northwestern University, who is lead author of a study involving almost 400,000 enrolled in lifestyle studies and followed for up to thirty years, is quoted as saying "I think these studies will wake people up and renew the emphasis on traditional risk factors."

---

13.   Sternberg, Steve. "Most Heart Attacks Caused by Unhealthy Lifestyle." *USA Today.* August 20, 2003: *SBC Yahoo News._News:_ http://www.Yahoo.com*

Most people know that diabetes can cause blindness, in addition to other problems. I believe it's easy to conclude that if walking at a fast pace three times a week for twenty minutes will prevent blindness, then making those walks a part of life should be easy. How can a person say to himself or herself, after blindness has set in, that the eyesight would still be there "If only I had taken those walks?"

A heart attack doesn't cause blindness, or the loss of a foot, arm, or some other visible body part. If a person survives, it's easy to believe life will go on and it won't happen again. But the heart attack kills a portion of the heart muscle. If that portion is just five percent, think of what it would look like on the outside of a person's body if five percent of that person's body was dead and everyone could see it every day. That five percent would cover half of a person's face.

Atrial fibrillation is a popular aspect of heart disease. An article entitled "Two Studies Point to Altered Approach on Atrial Fibrillation"[14] was published in *The New York Times*. The article said that atrial fibrillation is a common irregularity of the heartbeat that can lead to debilitating strokes and other life-threatening complications. "The studies being reported today in *The New England Journal of Medicine,* found that less costly and safer drugs that adjust the heart's rate, the speed at which it beats, are as effective as other drugs and procedures that control its rhythm, the regularity of that beat." The article continues "Until now, most American doctors have preferred a treatment strategy of restoring a normal heart rhythm, which can involve electrically shocking the heart, partly on the presumption that it lowered the incidence of complications like strokes more than with the heart-rate strategy. But the prevailing approach was largely uncontested, based on intuition rather than scientific study." The article lays the causes of atrial fibrillation as "heart attacks, heart failure, high blood pressure, damage to heart valves, diabetes, an overactive thyroid gland or excessive alcohol consumption. Sometimes, though, it occurs without any apparent underlying cause."

---

14. Falk, Rodney H. M.D., "Atrial Fibrillation." <u>The New England Journal of Medicine</u> Volume 344:1067-178, No. 14: 5 Apr. 2001.

Dr. Isadore Rosenfeld[15] writes that irregular heartbeats can be corrected permanently. Radio waves can correct these disturbances. A defibrillator wire can be threaded into the heart of a vulnerable individual and will shock the heart when it notices the beat is irregular. In his article, Dr. Rosenfeld says that the leading cause of sudden death in someone whose heart has been damaged by a heart attack is an unexpected life-threatening rhythm disorder, atrial fibrillation. Defibrillators, which shock and restore the normal heartbeat, come in compact, easy to use models. These compact models can be located in business offices and homes to be used by trained individuals.

Here's another article demonstrating the medical profession's progress in finding solutions to our health risks. The *San Jose Mercury News* published an article "In Profound Shift, Death Rates Drop for Heart Attack, Stroke", reported by Gina Kolata, in *The New York Times*.[16] Heart attack and strokes "remain the leading cause of death in the United States, but their toll is nothing like what it used to be. The typical heart-attack patient is no longer a man in his 50s who suddenly falls dead….Instead it is a man or woman of 70 or older, who survives." Dr. Claude Lenfant, director of the National Heart, Lung and Blood Institute said that now people can live another twenty or perhaps twenty-five years. But these older people are living with severe heart disease, and "These people aren't cured," said Dr. Eugene Braunwald, chief academic officer at Harvard Medical School's Partners Health Care System. The article goes on to say that "The plunging death rates have come about for an array of reasons—new drugs, new treatments, changes in behavior. No single change has made a huge difference, but the incremental advances have added up." Sixty-five percent of patients are reducing blood pressure with medication. When the article discusses death rates it is referring to deaths per thousand population. There are still a half million people dying from heart attacks every year, but our population has increased. Heart attacks are still way out in

---

15. Rosenfeld, Isadore, MD. "Why Cardiac Patients Can Take Heart." Parade Magazine. Feb 9, 2003: 8–10.

16. Kolata, Gina. "In profound shift, death rates drop for heart attack, stroke." The San Jose Mercury News. 19 Jan. 2003: A1+.

front, leading the pack, as the number one cause of death, premature or otherwise.

The other sources I've cited place heart attack deaths in the United States today at 500,000. The preceding article says that there would be 815,000 more deaths from heart attacks and 250,000 more deaths from stokes if medicine and personal behavior had not changed.

One final citation. Reporter Lisa M. Krieger[17] wrote about Mr. Viren Luther of Sunnyvale, California. Mr. Luther had a heart attack in 1979, at age forty-four. Ten years later he had a second attack. "He had four different pacemakers implanted, each replacing the last as medical technology advanced." At age sixty-eight, he was happy to be a doting grandfather. But look at the costs of treating heart problems. Published in the same article: Cholesterol drugs: $5,500 a year. Angioplasty: $19,000. Bypass surgery: $44,300. Heart transplant: $350,000. A heart transplant means someone else died to keep the recipient alive.

17.   Krieger, Lisa M., "Cardiac Strain." The San Jose Mercury News. 3 Sept. 2003. A1+

Part IV
My Recommendations

My wife, Dorothy, has patiently tolerated my exercise routine. It interferes with other family matters. Sometimes it appears as though the jogging is more important than my family. That certainly isn't true, but someone needs to walk in my shoes to understand my reasoning. I know that to be healthy I must eat right, get plenty of rest, and exercise. Does that sound familiar? Why is it that such simple advice is so difficult to follow?

COMMITMENT

Whoever is willing to begin exercising must make a *long-term commitment*. It shouldn't be tried for a couple of months or a couple of years. In a few weeks or months after stopping exercising a person loses whatever benefit that was gained and the short-term project will have a minor effect on a person's life. There is a benefit during the exercising time frame and for a short time thereafter, but the continuing benefits are lost in a surprisingly short time. Example; a person might live to age seventy-two without exercising. That person exercises for two years and then quits. That person can expect to live a few months longer than age seventy-two. I'm convinced it's possible life expectancy could be extended to perhaps age ninety-five or one hundred if that same person exercised continuously. What's more important is that that person will feel good, young, and healthy, right up to the end, whenever the end arrives.

PURPOSE

A major purpose of exercising is to cause oxygen to enter the lungs and blood stream. The continuous exercising (twenty minutes or longer) causes the oxygen to flow to all of the extremities of a person's body. It is my experience that fresh oxygen replaces stale oxygen. I am convinced this is what refreshes the body. The fresh oxygen doesn't reach the extremities if the blood pressure is allowed to be reduced during the process. If a person is jogging, swimming, biking, or engaged in some other routine in a stop and go manner, the fresh oxygen is forced part way towards the extremities and then backs up. Stop and go jogging means the fresh oxygen only goes part way, never all the way throughout the body. The fresh oxygen isn't allowed to replace all of the stale oxygen. Every form of exercising affects different muscles in the body. The common event in all exercising is the forcing of fresh oxygen into the body. My muscles relax when they've been sufficiently used, but my analysis of my own body has lead me to believe that the clear thinking and the feeling of being refreshed comes only from the fresh oxygen.

Exercising also builds the muscles of the body, including the heart muscle. The heart is a muscle, not an organ. There are many different kinds of cardiovascular exercise; swimming, rowing, biking, jogging, basketball, football, volley ball, tennis. A game or routine must be chosen that can be lived with. Tennis is good, so are basketball and rowing. Swimming is a great exercise. And walking is an excellent exercise. Just about anyone might enjoy walking. Walking has most of the oxygen benefits if the pace is fast and steady so as to raise the heart beat rate and keep it raised for at least twenty minutes. Walking needs to be done as a regular routine just as any other exercise. Anyone can walk in a mall or through a neighborhood. A person should start walking at a normal pace for the time and distance selected. The legs will ache, the hips will ache, the back muscles will ache, usually these muscles will ache at different times. This means muscles that have atrophied are now being used. Those muscles need to be coaxed back to life. One woman told me that her back muscles ached for six months.

After awhile it becomes easier to walk faster. And soon it's easier to walk farther in the same amount of time.

There are many books on running a person can read. Most of the books are geared towards turning a person into a runner, someone who runs hard for distance and speed. The books are geared towards competition and races. If some people want to prepare their bodies for racing, they should consider reading books authored by Bob Glover, Bill Rodgers, Joe Ellis, Lyle J. Michaly, M.D., and Dr. Cooper, of course. These authors can provide professional advice and guidance. If someone is jogging to stay alive, then there's no need for that person to be concerned with information explaining how to become competitive in the sport. But there's nothing to be lost by reading these authors' books.

As I've mentioned, I've never run a race since I began jogging, other than with my grandson, Rob Sabin. Rob was sixteen and an excellent 100-meter dash competitor in high school. Rob wanted to race so we agreed to go one time around the block. He'd never run three tenths of a mile. He was far ahead of me half way around the block, but he had to stop and walk the balance of the distance while I passed him. The next year he agreed to jog with me on my entire route. He stayed with me the full distance and finished ahead of me. That was the longest distance he'd ever run and he felt great having completed it on his first attempt. He learned that the distance run requires saving energy, rather than using it all up in the first few steps. When Rob was fifteen, his mother, Wendy, wanted him to challenge me in a push-up contest. Rob said he could do seventy-five. So I did seventy-five and then watched him as he did seventy-five. He didn't do seventy-six. (He might have stopped out of deference to my age.)

What about marathons and 10K races? Completing a marathon has nothing to do with my goals and objectives. Completing a marathon is a goal unto itself. My objective of controlling the health of my body is singular. I've watched others prepare for a marathon, complete the marathon, then stop exercising. It seems the strain on the body takes too much energy except for those athletes whose hearts and cardiovascular systems qualify them for physical superiority. A 10K race should not be a problem for me but the diversion is still contrary to my objective. 10K races are great for many people. If people use the 10K as a means of creating the exercise habit then it's even better. But if people make completing the race their sole objective, it serves no long-term purpose.

I would never take up jogging or running for the purpose of competing or just completing a race, the purpose would shortly come to an end. When I no longer believe I should exercise for the purpose of maintaining a healthy body and lifestyle, then my exercising will come to an end and soon I will come to an end.

Who takes up jogging when their reason is other than a health scare? Clarence "Bud" Ferrari, an attorney in San Jose began jogging several years before I started and was still jogging in 1992. T. J. Rodgers, President of Cypress Semiconductor in San Jose, told me that he started jogging when President John F. Kennedy advocated adopting a healthy lifestyle. He was still jogging in 1999. Dan Cheadle, Sr., who started and built a successful business, Cougar Components, Inc., in Sunnyvale, California has jogged for thirty years and still jogs at age 64. And my dentist, Dr. Lawrence Tottori, who jogged for over thirty years, but now walks and finds other forms of exercising to maintain his health. Dr. Tottori had heart problems, but never a heart attack. Others have begun and maintained jogging programs simply because they know it improves their health and clarifies their thinking process. Some people are quick to change to a new habit as soon as they recognize it will improve their well-being. All it takes is an explanation or a demonstration of the benefits.

Philosopher Alan Watts, who once held fellowships from Harvard University and the Bollinger Foundation, and was Episcopal Chaplain at Northwestern University during the Second World War, once said, "You don't sing to get to the end of the song." The same applies to my jogging. I don't jog to finish the jog. I don't jog to get it over with. I jog to stay alive and I like to do a little more than is required. The extra distance makes up for my slower pace, now that my speed is diminishing.

HEART

What happens when a person has a heart attack? The amount of damage to the heart will determine life or death. The amount of scar tissue also determines the amount of strain the heart can tolerate thereafter. Here's how I learned about this limitation. My wife and I were in Eugene, Oregon, visiting our daughter, Wendy, her husband and children in 1998. Her then husband, Doug, likes to ride bikes, so he and their daughter, Rachel, and I rode bikes around town and by the Willamette River. We went down an embankment off the road and onto a dirt trail. There was a short but steep drop down to the trail. When we returned we had to ride back up the embankment. I tried to ride the bike up the incline and my breathing stopped as I pushed hard on the bike pedals. That strain was just too much for my heart. I learned very quickly why a doctor must monitor a person's exercise routine after the person has a heart attack. My normal exercising routine is a habit that doesn't challenge the heart muscle. The undamaged part of the heart is very strong and performs quite well, but it has its limits. I talked to Dr. Siegel about eliminating the damage caused by the heart attacks through my exercise program. He told me that was impossible.

My ability to incur a sudden outburst of strength and speed is gone forever. It's been my opinion that creating new muscle fiber or tissue on the heart (if that is possible) would allow a person to increase his or her capacity, but it wouldn't allow the person to compete in the same manner as someone whose heart is not damaged. Because I've learned to pace the use of my energy, I can perform physical activities and work better than most people much younger. It's the same with my exercising. I can keep going at a steady, hard pace, but I can't go to the extreme that would be required to win a race.

If a person has had a heart attack, that person must find his or her limits and stay within those limits. Always be guided by a physician. A person can increase the strength of the other muscles in the body, which increases the physical exertion capacity without increasing the exertion on the heart beyond its capacity. In return, that will increase the strength of the heart, which will make it easier to force fresh oxygen through the body.

In 2000, Dr. Siegel decided to complete an echocardiogram because my stamina is so high, and he wanted to check my heart with more than just the ECG and treadmill. The procedure is to complete the treadmill exam, lie down on a table, then immediately complete the echocardiogram. The echocardiogram allows the operator and the doctor to see the heart. This made it easier for him to locate the scar tissue.

It has been my experience that heart disease was not debilitating after I began and sustained an exercise program. Thirty years without medication after the discovery of my heart disease seems to me to be quite remarkable, not because it is me, but because it can be done. Other than six months use of coumadin, I was medication free for thirty-five years.

CANCER

I do contract carcinomas when I jog in the sunlight. Wearing a hat protects me to some degree, but Dr. Leon Lubianker in Los Gatos has removed all of the spots before they became serious. I developed cancer on my right ear in 2002, and Dr. Lubianker referred me to Dr. Greg Morganroth in Mountain View who was able to remove the cancer without any serious complications.

TENSION

Tension and stress are good things to discuss right now. I've had to deal with as much stress as anyone. The fact that I've always seemed to be pulling and tearing muscles is a good measurement of the stress I've felt from time to time. When my body is tense at the beginning of my jog, it is always without the tension at the end of my jog. Sometimes I've traded a pulled muscle for the tension; nevertheless, the tension is gone. That's a good trade-off. But it's taken many years for me to learn there is no need for a trade-off. When I am tense, all I've needed to do is slow down a little bit and jog a few more minutes.

Our muscles consist of at least two sets. One is the viscera (smooth internal muscles) and the other the striated muscles (outer muscles). When we become tense the visceral muscles will tighten along with the striated muscles. The striated muscles will relax quickly but the visceral muscles need many hours to relax. In my body, the visceral muscles begin to relax as they warm up from the body heat while jogging. That's why exercising releases my tension. When the muscles relax, the tension relaxes.

Too many disappointments could have caused me to stop my program. Too many conflicts could have caused me stop any exercise program. The reasons to quit are myriad. I can have a nasty argument with my wife. My marriage might break up. I can get involved in a lawsuit. I can have conflicts at work, lose my job, go without income for long periods of time. My expenses can increase, and my income can go down. Cars can try to hit me. Other people at the facilities can get in my way. Pulled muscles, torn knees, shin splints, torn tendons, and heart problems could discourage me. I could use any of these reasons to destroy my health. I could even lose a leg. (I've never lost a leg, thank God, but I did watch a man in Anderson, Indiana with one leg and a prosthesis jog for several miles.)

There have been many difficulties in my family's life that could have been used as an excuse to quit exercising. By moving to Indiana, I began a business and a personal odyssey that wreaked havoc on me and my family. Business and personal difficulties caused me to change my entire method of earning a living. Legal problems that should have lasted one or two years continued for fourteen years. The strain on our marriage caused my wife and I to separate after living in Indiana for ten years. That separation lasted for six years. We reunited in Santa Clara, California. The jogging and resistance exercising made it possible for me to survive the turmoil. If I had not created the exercise habit, and if I had not died by age forty, then I surely would have been dead by age forty-five.

Many people tell me they don't jog because it's boring. That depends on a person's goals and objectives. If a person likes to race cars or raise hell with the neighbors, then jogging is boring compared to those actions. But jogging is more exciting than death or failing health or the inability to get off the couch. To me, staying alive isn't boring. And I'm certainly not looking for excitement while jogging. If I want excitement, I can always throw a rock through my neighbor's window. Then my jogging might come in handy, temporarily. If a person is bored, that person isn't exerting the body—boredom and exhaustion don't go hand-in-hand.

CONTROL

Many exercises require partners or facilities. Facilities are not always available to accommodate the schedule of someone who exercises regularly. Relying on a partner or a team can create disappointments. The partner or team might not be able to get together on schedule. They might not have the same commitment.

A person is in absolute control of the jogging and walking exercise schedule and routine when it is done alone. The hours can change, the route, the city, the clothes, everything that goes into jogging or walking can be accommodated. If a person wants to maintain control, then that person should select jogging or walking. If jogging is selected, walking should be tried first.

It's pretty easy to change from walking to jogging if the proper shoes are worn. All that is needed is to walk for a distance, then jog ten paces, walk for another distance and jog another ten paces. Soon the jog can be increased to fifteen paces, eventually twenty paces. Jogging becomes the order of the day pretty quickly. It isn't necessary to become a jogger, but this will work. Jogging will do a much better job of forcing oxygen out to the extremities of a body. A person also needs to know the condition of his or her heart. If the heart is weak, its strength can be gradually increased. The strength of a heart can be built up slowly, just as any other muscle in the body. Remember how long it took me to build up the strength in my arms and shoulders when doing the bench press? And it took me two years to build up my heart muscle so that I could jog two miles steady. A person should build the muscles up to a certain level, stay there for awhile, then build them up a little more. There's no reason to rush it.

I prefer jogging counterclockwise, although I'm convinced this preference is a habit just as any other habit. Nature might support my position on this habit. The Earth spins counterclockwise, it rotates around the Sun in a counterclockwise direction, and our Solar System moves through space in a counterclockwise direction. A counterclockwise direction for jogging makes sense to me.

I've jogged on cushioned tracks, cement, tar, dirt, cinder, just about every kind of surface. The surface has never made any difference to me. Some joggers have told me that a hard jogging surface gave them shin splints. I have my own theory on shin splints. When jogging, my foot needs to land on the heel, roll onto my toes, and then my foot leaves the ground. If I try to jog by running on the balls of my feet, I'll tear muscles and exhaust myself very quickly. Running on the balls of my feet is for sprinting. If I jog flat footed, it has the effect of jamming the foot onto the surface. Jogging flat footed could cause shin splints. Nothing should be forced. A nice, smooth, rolling pace has never caused problems for my feet or shins. The best pace for jogging is a pace where I must exert myself. I start out slowly and let the body warm up before hitting my normal pace.

I'm a pedestrian and belong on the sidewalk. I need to be careful because of outdoor obstacles. Trees and bushes are allowed to grow out over the sidewalk. Once or twice a year I'll traverse the jogging route and trim the foliage so the branches won't poke out an eye or the barbs won't scratch my body or tear my clothes. No property owner has ever complained. Another obstacle is the automobile. I have jogged in the street in competition with the cars, but each time it was a mistake on my part. Sometimes I'm forced into the street. If a sidewalk is blocked by a car, I must use the street. When I come to an intersection I nearly always pay deference to the auto. I'll always lose a contest between myself and a car or truck. I'll jog a few extra feet along the sidewalk until I'm behind the cars, then jog in back of them as I cross the street. When I'm jogging outside, I'll pass driveways and cross intersections. It's important to remember that auto drivers usually look only in the direction of traffic before proceeding. I can be within one or two feet of the auto and the driver may not see me. I need to look directly into the eyes of the driver, and if he or she doesn't notice me, then I either stop and wait or jog behind the auto. Some drivers are very courteous and will defer to the jogger. Other drivers believe its up to the jogger to get out of the way.

On December 17, 2002, Because of the weather and traffic, I was walking across the intersection at Blossom Hill Road and Beswick, on the north side of the street in front of the entrance and exit to the Magic Sands mobile home compound. It was still dark outside and raining, but the intersection is very well lit so that it resembles daylight. A car pulled into the crosswalk area and stopped for the red semaphore. I had the green light, so I began walking across in front of the car. I reached the headlamp on the driver's side of the car when the car started forward and turned right. The car pushed me so that I stumbled and ran for about fifteen feet, trying to keep from falling on my face. I stopped my fall with my hands on the ground, turned around and called to the driver. The car stopped, the driver saw that I was vertical and then sped off.

Things can block a sidewalk. One day a garbage can was placed on the sidewalk and I tried to jog around it. My foot hit the edge of the curb and I slid down the street on my body. That left some solid scrapes on my legs and arms. Another time a neighbor had installed a new roof. The contractor placed his advertising sign in the middle of the sidewalk. I was jogging at about 6:00 AM, and it was still dark outside. I came around the corner, hit the sign, and slid down the sidewalk on my leg. The slide took a large chunk of skin out of my upper thigh and left large tears on my knee and lower leg. I put the sign on my neighbor's lawn. Two days later the sign was back on the sidewalk. This time I walked back to my neighbor's house and showed him the damage to my body. The sign was gone the next time I jogged. It didn't affect my jogging routine but it took about a month to heal.

Again, on February 11, 2003, I was jogging down Blossom Hill Road and came to the Beswick intersection at about 6:25 AM. The sidewalk crossing was blocked because the city had been repairing that section, so I stepped out into the street and crossed the intersection, then continued on my route. I reached the same spot the second time around the loop, but this time when I jogged out to the street I stepped into wet cement. A worker had begun laying new cement around the underground utility stations. He was in the process of laying cement just around the corner and had dumped the excess cement in the dirt area between the sidewalk and the street. I moved towards the street to avoid the wet cement sidewalk and stepped right into the middle of the cement puddle. When I stepped into the cement my legs started to fly out from under me. I could have fallen onto the curb if I wasn't able to catch my balance. I assume he didn't expect anyone to walk by at that time of day.

There are other interferences. When I jog for any distance it stimulates my bowels. I had to find a solution to carrying toilet paper. The distance around the block we live on is three tenths of a mile. I do my morning stretching exercises, then jog twice around the block. I return to the house and use the bathroom. This works and lets me concentrate on my jog. This wasn't a problem when jogging at a Y or sports club. I could just leave the track and return. But having my bowels act up can be embarrassing when jogging around a neighborhood of single family dwellings and apartment units.

I've read articles detailing what a person should think about while jogging. I've seen joggers wearing earphones and listening to a cassette tape. Wearing earphones will isolate the jogger from the environment. Concentrating on the cassette tape interferes with noticing the occurrence of surrounding events and prevents the jogger from recognizing the immediate effect jogging has on the body. If a person is moving at a pace that takes effort, that person needs to know how it affects the body. The jogger also needs to be keenly aware of the environment, a miscue can be dangerous. I've never worn earphones or other means of distractions. My thoughts are almost exclusively on what is happening around me and to me. The jog is a vitally important part of my life. Those few minutes are what keep me alive and healthy so I don't want to treat them lightly or give them short shrift. I concentrate on the here and now, this moment in time.

I took up jogging to stay alive. There could be other reasons for other people, but staying alive was my primary reason. The length of time I jog and the distance I cover are my friends. They give me health, energy, and life. I need the time and the distance; I've learned not to rush them. I've set my goals. I need to maintain my exercise routine to maintain my health. I'm convinced that once committed to maintaining a long and healthy life, exercising must be a lifetime routine. I committed myself to five years because that was two years longer than my life expectancy. After five years the habit was strong but so was the desire to continue living. What I did to stay alive worked. I decided to continue doing what worked. Why should I trade known success for possible failure? The key to developing a healthy body is a decision, commitment, and discipline. It's a combined mental and physical commitment. The decision was one where I forced my mind to take control of my brain and body.

I couldn't jog slowly for a tenth of a mile when I first began to jog. Two years later I could jog two miles, although at quite a slow pace. At three years my pace was about eight minutes per mile, for two miles. At five years my pace was 7'15" per mile. My pace leveled off at about 7'30" until my eighteenth year. It slowly increased to eight minutes over the next three years. My pace was dramatically affected by the heart muscle events. But after the heart attacks, my pace picked up and I could easily jog three miles after the first angioplasty and my pace and distance weren't affected very much. But then, the length of time it took me to travel my distance continued to increase. The most dramatic increase and change in my jogging time has happened after reaching age seventy.

Early morning stretching exercises are just that, to stretch. The total time required is six minutes. It wakes me up and sets the tone for the day. Stretching before jogging is recommended by many authors, but I have never considered it to be essential.

From June 9, 1992, until January 16, 1997, I recorded sunrise every jogging day. From January 19, 1997, until May 20, 1999, I kept track of both sunrise and sunset. It gave me perspective on the symmetry of the Sun and the Earth. The sunrise information helped me pay closer attention to the movement of the sun. It covers a vast distance from north to south. From November 16, 1992, until May 20, 1999, I kept track of the temperature and weather conditions. The temperature and weather move in symmetry, too.

COURTESY

How about courtesy or diplomacy while jogging? An issue that comes up on jogging tracks is who's on the inside and who's on the outside of the track. Some joggers want the inside of the track and ask those who are walking to use the outside of the track. Others prefer to have the walkers use the inside of the track. Those who walk seldom walk alone. The controversy comes up because walkers seem to need someone with them for conversational purposes. When two, three, or four people are trying to walk abreast so they can all be included in the same conversation it creates a traffic block. If there are more than two persons, they need to walk abreast because it is difficult for their voices to carry from front to back, and vice versa, while moving fairly quickly at a steady pace. It makes it very difficult for the joggers to get past the walkers when this happens on a small track. If a six foot wide track is slanted, those walking or jogging side by side can cause real traffic problems. It forces other joggers to constantly slow down and speed up every time they reach two or more walkers in a group. Most joggers use a clock or watch as a measuring device to control their time and distance and when they need to find a way to pass walkers who are blocking their path, it causes them to lose the flow of their pace.

EQUIPMENT

What equipment did I need to get started? I started with just a pair of gym shoes, shorts, and a T-shirt. After a couple of years I switched to jogging shoes. I own at least two pair of jogging shoes so that I can change shoes and socks after the jog. Changing shoes and socks reduces the possibility of fungus growth between my toes and on my feet. I need shorts and a T shirt for summer. Women will need a sports bra. I wear a cap. I need heavier clothes for colder weather. The temperature in San Jose ranges from a low of around 28° in the winter to a high of 100° in the summer. At 6:00 AM the temperature is usually around 35° in the winter and 60° in the summer. When the temperature drops below 40°, I wear a wool cap and white garden gloves. I also wear a heavier sweat shirt over the T-shirt and long sweat pants. I try to find clothing that will be comfortable for about two thirds of the distance of my jog. The proper amount of clothing is a trial and error process.

<u>USING WEIGHTS.</u> I try to use weights so that the muscles being worked receive maximum benefit. I use the amount of weights for each exercise that my muscles can handle without using other muscles as an aid. For example, I keep my legs flat on the bench when I'm doing the bench press. If I bend my knees with my feet on the bench then I'll press with my legs to force the weights up in the air. This arches my back. The eventual result is either a pulled back muscle or a strained leg muscle. Instead, I can add or subtract weight when I concentrate on the particular muscles I'm trying to work. Using individual free weights works different muscles than using both hands and arms to manipulate the weights on a single bar. I noticed that I became exhausted and the exhaustion remained the entire day when I used more weight and more repetitions. I adjusted the weights to create a feeling of freshness during the balance of the day.

WEATHER

Moving to California was really a godsend for me, because I became used to jogging outside. I can set my own schedule without concern over facilities. The weather allows for outside jogging twelve months of the year. The weather and the amount of clothing I wear seems to have a minor effect on me, my time, and my distance. My jogging time does increase in the winter because of the extra weight of the clothing. I've found the best temperature to be between 58° and 62°. In that temperature range, sun or rain, it's really nice to jog. Everything feels just great.

I've jogged in many states and cities. In Florida, the humidity slowed me down and made it harder for me to breathe. Still I would find an area where I could jog and find my way back to the motel. In Phoenix, Arizona, I would jog down one side of the street on the sidewalk for twenty minutes, cross over the street at an intersection and jog back. I've done the same in Los Angeles. In Eugene, Oregon, visiting our daughter, her husband and children, I'd jog from the Red Lion Motel down to the Willamette River, along the river and then across the river on a bridge, turn around and return to the motel. I wasn't able to measure the distance in these situations, so I'd jog for around forty-five minutes. Salt Lake City, Utah, had an excellent gymnasium downtown which was owned by the Church of Jesus Christ of Latter-day Saints (Mormon). It had a jogging track, basketball court, handball courts, weight rooms, swimming pools, showers, and just about every health club utility. I've used that facility many times even though I'm not a Mormon. It was torn down and replaced with a convention center, and that forced me out on the streets of the neighborhood wherever I happened to be staying. In Salt Lake City, I'd either find a high school and use the track, or I'd jog around the neighborhood just like in the other cities. Jogging three and one-half to four miles in Salt Lake City is a real struggle for me. The city is located at a high altitude, and it's on the side of a mountain. Jogging around the neighborhood usually means jogging up and down hills. The hilly terrain and the altitude really make it tough.

Sometimes it rains. What to do in the rain? I jog. The clothing gets wet, but the heat generated from jogging keeps me warm in rainy, cool weather. The rain feels good in warm weather. In any event, I find it's fun to jog in the rain. I've jogged in snow only a few times. It seldom snows in Salem, Oregon. I've never seen it snow in San Jose. It snows a lot in the Midwest. Indiana has very cold, snowy weather in the winter. Nearly every YMCA in Indiana has a jogging track but sometimes they are closed for repairs and maintenance. Those few times the Y's or spas were closed forced me to jog outside in the snow and cold. I just put on warmer clothes and jogged around the neighborhood. I've been asked why I jog in the rain, snow, with pulled muscles, or if it interferes with other important activities. I jog to stay alive, not as a convenience. I don't get a high from jogging and it's not a thrill. If there is something happening which seems more important than my jogging then it must be more important than my staying alive. If it's that important, my presence will have no effect.

SLEEP

Getting plenty of sleep is important. I make sure I get eight hours each night and, if not, then I make up for lost sleep within a day or two or take a nap during the day. I have heard it said from reliable medical sources (sorry, I don't have them at my fingertips) that you cannot make up for lost sleep. Since I've jogged early in the morning for the last thirteen years, that means I usually get up around 5:30 AM. It also means I must go to bed at 9:30 PM. And it means that television has become less important in my life. One night I went to bed about 1:00 AM and got up at 5:30 AM on schedule. I dressed to jog and jogged about a mile before I knew what I was doing. It seemed like I woke up at the mile mark. Recently, lack of sleep has also been connected with weight gain. Just Google "lost sleep" and you will get numerous hits.

ILLNESS AND HEALTH

I seem to escape most illnesses, and I've never been prone to depression, for which I'm grateful. I believe the fresh oxygen that passes through my body is the most potent elixir on the planet. I believe oxygen cures illnesses and cleanses the brain. There's no substitute for fresh oxygen and no better method of self-administration. From time to time, I'll catch a cold just like everyone else. I jog when I have a cold and I've jogged when I had flu. These illnesses don't seem to slow me down very much. The jogging does give me temporary relief. The flu has less of a deleterious effect on me, and I think that's because my body heat helps kill some of the virus. This is only conjecture. I've been administered flu shots every year since I reached age sixty-five, and that helps avoid the flu. Colds are next to impossible to beat. Perhaps some day the medical profession will eradicate the common cold just as it has smallpox.

AGE

What role does age play in an exercising program? Not much. (I'm not comparing an exercise program to competition. Age makes a big difference in competition.) I'll concede that nursing home residents are not candidates for long term exercising programs, but there are very few people whose health has deteriorated below the state of my health in the fall of 1967. I started exercising when I knew it was the best alternative for me. But is it necessary for someone to wait until that person's health is as bad as mine? It might be a lot smarter to begin an exercise program while still healthy.

How to Eat

That's easy, right? Just put food in my mouth, chew, and swallow. I really don't need to chew, just swallow. When my daughters were very young, I told them they could put the food under their armpits and squeeze. What about food? A few years ago I read a newspaper item that said people eat on average seventeen times a day. That means some people eat more than seventeen times a day and some people eat less than seventeen times a day. It also means that most people eat without knowing they are eating—they do it unconsciously. I've never kept a log of everything I've consumed, it's too cumbersome. I've used a different method. Eating right is something that I learned when I was paying attention to what I was consuming. I always believed that I knew just how much I was eating and when I ate it. But I was eating out of habit and eating unconsciously. As a result, I was eating many times a day.

I gained control of my weight by eating only at set times during the day. In the beginning, that meant eating something every two hours. After a few months I knew from habit what I took into my body. Now I eat five times a day. I eat breakfast, lunch, snack, dinner, and another snack. My snacks consist of fruits and nuts. Most fruits are very delicious. The fruits also help with digestion. Once that habit was established, I started to skip one eating period several times a week. Skipping that small amount of food brought my weight down very slowly. Skipping a meal, usually lunch or the snack at night, would cause me to be hungry. My stomach demanded to be filled up. There were times I could have eaten a board. But I would not give in and waited until the next mealtime arrived. Now I know exactly what I eat and when I eat it. I eat chicken, turkey, or fish. And I eat fresh fruits every day. I eat two fruits at breakfast, a grapefruit and a banana. I'll usually eat three fruits a day, but sometimes I'll eat four or five fruits. I also eat nuts; peanuts, walnuts, pistachios, and cashews. When I need to lose a pound or two I'll eat breakfast late and skip lunch. But going without food for more than six hours will stretch my limits. I become a little testy after six hours without food during the day. If I eat at 10 AM, then I need to eat a snack sometime between 10 AM and 6 PM. While I'm in the process of exercising, it keeps my mind off food and allows me to eat a generous portion when I do eat.

I don't believe the stomach is a muscle. It doesn't expand and contract like a muscle, it stretches. My belief is that if the size of the stomach is to be reduced, it must atrophy. When I skip a meal and have hunger pangs, the stomach is in the process of atrophying. When I reduce food intake, the stomach must shrink to eliminate hunger pangs and that takes time. I've never tried to lose a lot of weight in a hurry. Losing thirty to forty pounds over a two- to five-year period of time is plenty fast. It should be done slowly. I've met many people who would like to decrease their weight from perhaps 225 pounds to perhaps 160 pounds in three months, but I've never met anyone whose weight increased from 160 pounds to 225 pounds in three months. Going both directions takes time. Losing weight is easy when following this pattern.

I have weighed myself every day since 1967. My weight loss was so slow that no one has ever asked me how I lost my weight. The comments I've received have been about how I've never had to worry about gaining weight. People, even family members, think of me as having always been slim. When my body was too heavy, it was impossible to maintain the jog for the required twenty minutes. Losing weight made jogging easier. When I maintained an exercise program with a constant level of energy output for a set period of time I developed a lean body, because a lean body made it easier for me to accomplish my goal.

Sometimes I'll go for several years without eating sugar and a minimum of salt. Then I'll eat sugar and salt for a while. If I'm studying or learning new material, the sugar seems to help me remember what I read. At the same time, the sugar puts extra pounds on my body. When I eat sugar, I cut back on other foods to maintain a level intake. I used to eat a lot of chocolate and drink a lot of coffee, but I don't do that anymore. Coffee and chocolate are stimulants that can initiate an irregular heart beat.

Part V
<u>CONCLUSION</u>

After I had completed thirty years of jogging and resistance exercising. I traveled back to Salem, Oregon, and met with my friend, Dr. Harmon Harvey, and thanked him for alerting me to my serious health problem. His warning motivated me to take positive action to correct a decrepit body. I thanked him for keeping me alive.

Some people would consider five years as a very long commitment, and that might be true. Yet, it is a very short time in retrospect. Five years is less than one-seventh of thirty-seven years. The thirty-seven years have passed very rapidly. In September 2003, I was seventy-two. In November 2004 I reached age seventy-four. That means I've lived the last half of my life following a dedicated exercise routine. The second half of my life has certainly been more rewarding than the first half. Remember the Bee Gees, "Staying Alive."

I intend to keep a record of my exercising for the rest of my life. But there comes a time when it's best to finish the book and let someone else read how my exercising has affected my staying alive. It has reached that point for me. The process of maintaining my health and staying alive is very much a routine, and it's easy. And for anyone else, all a person needs to do is walk for twenty minutes, five days a week. A steady walk at a decent pace. Don't walk the dog or stop to smell the flowers. Keep going so that the oxygen flows all the way through the body. It's the fresh oxygen that cleanses the body, cures illnesses, and refreshes the mind. A two mile walk is better, but the twenty minutes will do the job. If anyone suffers from heart disease, diabetes, depression, or any other illness, then that person needs to take a walk on a regular basis and begin increasing his/her exercising. Anyone can take charge of his own body and let the doctor help when needed, rather than expecting the doctor to repair or cure the damage when the body goes uncared for.

There are parts of this book that are routine reading and perhaps not very interesting to many people. However, if staying alive well beyond a scheduled date of death is exciting, then the entire book is exciting. Developing a routine that keeps the body healthy and then maintaining that routine forever (forever meaning for as long as a person lives) is the key to health. Firecrackers don't go off, the press doesn't come around and write stories and take pictures, crowds don't gather and cheer, no medals are given. When a person stays alive longer than that person should have lived, it gives that person more time to contribute to the welfare of that person's family, friends, and society as a whole. Staying alive isn't selfish, it's contributory. One of the nice things about committing suicide is that most people don't know they're doing it. People don't notice the changes in their bodies from day to day. Me, I've learned how to keep my body alive. I've have some bad years, but if I stick around long enough there will always be good years ahead.

My doctor said I had three years to live over thirty-seven years ago. When I took charge of my own body and health I was able to expand that three years to more than twelve times as long, and I'm still going strong. I suggest that everyone take primary control over their own bodies and health and treat those bodies like temples.

Part VI
Statistics

For those who like statistics, I'm going to provide some of the data from my ledger. I'll list my jogging times twice a year from 1991 to March 30, 1999. Then the times are listed for the last jog of each month from August 1999 until December 2004. I'll also list the times just before and after my hernia operation, the first episode of atrial fibrillation (which was short-lived), and just before and after my last atrial fibrillation and an episode of nonsustained ventricular tachycardia.

		Time	Time	
Year	Distance	March 30	September 30	(closest date)
1991	3.15 miles	27'57"	27'05"	Age 60
1992		26'28"	25'47"	
1993		26'20"	26'26"	
1994		27'26"	27'26"	
1995		27'23"	27'37"	
1996		27'01"	27'27"	
1997		28'19"	28'40"	
1998		29'25"	29'27"	
1999		30'15"	32'59"	

		End of Each Month	
Year	Distance	Month	Time
1999	3.4 miles	August	34'26"
		September	32'59"

		October	34'25"	
		November	35'38"	Age 69
		December	35'04"	
2000		January	35'10"	
		February	34'49"	
		March	33'04"	
		April	33'39"	
	4 miles	May	41'53"	In Salt Lake City
		June	34'29"	
		July	33'11"	
		August	35'29"	
		September	35'54"	
		October	34'45"	
		November	34'44"	Age 70
		December	33'46"	
2001		January	34'38"	
		February	34'41"	
		March	34'47"	
		April	35'18"	
		May	36'00"	
		June	35'25"	
	4 miles	July	44'40"	In Salt Lake City
	longer than 4 miles	August	52'09"	In Eugene, Oregon
		September	35'58"	
		October	36'03"	
		November	35'34"	Age 71
		December	35'38"	
2002		January	36'26"	

		February	35′40″	
		March	37′27″	
		April	35′06″	
		May	36′25″	
		June	35′47″	
		July	35′47″	
	longer than 4 miles	August	45′12″	In Salt Lake City
		September	36′31″	
		October 15th	ventricular tachycardia and atrial fibrillation	
		October	43′56″	
		November	41′01″	Age 72
		December	48′14″	
2003	3.4 miles	January	40′01″	
		February	38′25″	
		March	39′32″	
		April	40′57″	
		May	39′42″	
		June	41′12″	
		July	39′13″	
		August	39′56″	
		September	40′21″	
		October	41′04″	
		November	41′16″	Age 73
		December	42′47″	
2004		January	39′48″	
		February	40′39″	
		March	41′31″	
		April	40′07″	

	May	39'17"	
	June	39'52"	
	July	40'29"	
	August	44'31"	sore left rib muscle
	September	40'41"	
	October	40'58"	
2.2 miles	November	28'46"	
	December	28'43"	

Hernia operation:

2/6/97	3.15 miles	28'22"	
2/9/97		28'24"	
2/11/97		28'02"	
2/13/97		29'09"	
2/14/97		operation	
2/18/97		57'33"	walked
2/20/97		55'45"	walked
2/23/97		52'28"	walked
2/25/97		38'58"	walked and jogged
2/29/97		29'50"	jogged

First atrial fibrillation event (this happened just as I completed 30 years of jogging):

8/31/97	3.15 miles	28'57"	
9/2/97		29'52"	
9/4/97		29'16"	
9/7/97		29'42"	
9/9/97		Did not finish, atrial fibrillation. Stopped and walked several times.	

9/13/97	3.15	did not time	walked
9/14/97		did not time	walked
9/16/97		did not time	walked
9/18/97		did not time	walked
9/21/97	3.15	28′56″	jogged
9/23/97		29′15″	jogged
9/25/97		29′41″	jogged
9/28/97		28′40″	jogged

Atrial fibrillation, an episode of nonsustained ventricular tachycardia (October 15, 2002):

10/5/02	3.4 miles	35′28″	jogged
10/8/02		36′06″	jogged
10/10/02		36′21″	jogged
10/12/02		39′05″	jogged
10/15/02	ventricular tachy-cardia atrial fibril-lation	42′18″	stopped and walked three times
10/17/02		47′46″	jogged
10/19/02		53′57″	walked
10/22/02		53′15″	walked
10/24/02		51′51	walked
10/26/02		49′15″	walked
10/29/02		42′04″	slow jog
10/31/02		43′55″	slow jog
11/2/02		41′50″	slow jog until 12/10/02
12/10/02		44′05″	slow jog, very exhausting
12/12/02		52′11″	walked until 1/16/03
1/9/03		47′08″	walk
1/11/03		46′24″	walk
1/14/03		46′33″	walk

1/15/03	stress test and echocardiogram	
1/16/03	46'23"	Walk, but slow jog 100 paces five times during last one-half mile. Seemed to breathe stale air for about 15 minutes afterwards.
1/18/03	45'25"	Same as 1/16/03, but I didn't feel any stale air.
1/21/03	45'05"	Walked, jogged 150 paces Four times last one-half mile. No stale air.
1/23/03	45'08"	Walked, jogged the last mile slowly. No stale air.
1/25/03	39'46"	Jogged and walked intermittently. Jog 1/4th mile, walk 1/8th mile. No feelings of stale air.
5/31/03	39'42"	Reduced the dosage of beta blocker to 50 mg. 5/24/03 and my head became clearer. I'm beginning to feel more normal although my speed is still quite slow.

| 6/12/03 | 37'33" | Felt good. |
| 6/21/03 | 41'43" | Tendon in my foot and cortisone. |

Here's a partial history of my body weight on March 30 and September 30:

Year	March 30	September 30 (closest date)
1991	170	166
1992	165	160
1993	163	161
1994	158	156
1995	156	159
1996	161	163
1997	161	161
1998	160	160
1999	160	161
2000	160	160
2001	162	160
2002	160	160
2003	164	162

Here's a partial history of the weight exercises as recorded in my journal.

On August 17, 1993	Weights	Repetitions	Sets
Power push-ups		60	1
Arm curls	25	10	3
Arm curls	45	10	4
Forearm lift	25	10	1
Bench press	130	25	1
Bench press	140	20	1
Bench press	140	15	1

| Bench press | 140 | 12 | 1 |
| Back arm dips | 35 | 1 | 1 |

On June 30, 1994

Power push-ups	body weight	60	1
Arm curls	25	10	3
Arm curls	45	10	4
Forearm lift	25	10	1
Bench press	130	25	1
Bench press	140	15	1
Bench press	140	12	1
Bench press	140	7	1
Back arm dips		35	1

August 7, 1994

Power push-ups		64	1
Arm curls	25	12	2
Arm curls	35	12	2
Forearm lift	25	10	1
Bench press	130	20	1
Bench press	140	18	1
Bench press	140	16	1
Back arm dips		36	1

September 9, 1997

Power push-ups		64	1
Arm curls	25	12	2
Arm curls	45	12	2
Forearm lift	25	10	1
Bench press	140	18	1

Bench press	140	16	1
Bench press	140	14	1
Back arm dips		35	1

March 11, 1999

Power push-ups		64	1
Arm curls	25	12	2
Arm curls	35	12	2
Forearm lift	25	10	1
Bench press	130	18	1
Bench press	130	16	1
Bench press	130	14	1
Back arm dips		35	1

December 17, 2002

Power push-ups		50	1
Arm curls	25	10	4
Forearm lift	25	10	1
Bench press	110	10	1
Bench press	110	10	1
Back arm dips		25	1

July 1, 2003

Power push-ups		50	1
Arm curls	25	10	4
Forearm lift	25	10	1
Bench press	110	10	1
Bench press	120	10	1
Bench press	130	10	1
Back arm dips		25	1

<u>December 31, 2003</u>

Power push-ups		50	1
Arm curls	25	10	4
Forearm lift	25	10	1
Bench press	110	14	1
Bench press	120	12	1
Bench press	130	12	1
Back arm dips		25	1

Some medical data on September 9, 1999:

Cholesterol was	178
TRI	52
LDL	125
HDL	43

<u>Here's a listing of some of my medical data as of March 4, 2003:</u>

BMP		
LYTES	NA	142
K	4.1	
CL	105	
CO2	30	
GLU	91	
BUN	28	High
CREAT	1.2	
CA	8.7	
PT		
PT	13.8	High
INR	1.2	
CBC		

Hemogram		
WBC	6.9	
RBC	4.6	
HGB	14.9	
HCT	43	
MCV	93	
MCH	32	
MCHC	35	
RDW	12.8	
PLT	173	
NEUT %	69	
LYMP %	23	
MONO %	8	
EOS %	0	
BASO %	0	

Lipids

Cholesterol	210	High {100-199}
Triglycerides	159	High {0-144}
VLDL	32	{5-35}
LDL Cholesterol	141	High {0-129}
HDL Cholesterol	37	Low {> 39}
Cholesterol/hdl Ratio	5.7 Average Risk Factor	
LDL/HDL Ratio	3.82	

Coagulation

Prothrombin	34.4

CBC platelets and comprehensive metabolic panel numbers were within range, except for urea nitrogen which was 27. Magnesium was within range, but thyroid stimulating hormone (TSH) was below range at 18.

Works Cited

Altman, Lawrence K. "Two Studies Point to Altered Approach on Atrial Fibrillation." *The New York Times.* December 5, 2000: A41

American Heart Association: http://www.americanheart. org/presenter.jhtml?identifier=4591. 21 June 2005

Blackman, H. "Personality and Mood of Former Elite Male Athletes-A Descriptive Study." International Journal of Sports Medicine, Vol.22, April 2001: 215-220.

Brigham and Women's Hospital, Boston, Reuters. "Study Links Sleep Imbalance to Heart Attacks." Archives of Internal Medicine (January 2003) *Yahoo News.* Http://www.yahoo.com. January 27, 2003.

Burfoot, Amy. *Runner's World Complete Book of Running.* Emmas, PA: Rodale Press, Inc. 1977.

Caruso, David B. "Overweight Adults Die Three Years Sooner, Study Finds." *San Jose Mercury News.* January 7, 2003: A7. From AP News Service.

Cassidy, Mike. "Runner Seeing Double." *San Jose Mercury News.* October 22, 2001: B1+.

Cooper, Kenneth, M.D., M.P.H. *Aerobics.* New York: Bantam, 1968.

"Exercise for the Mind." *Reader's Digest.* Mar. 2000: 44 (Condensed from article in *Psychology Today)*

Falk, Rodney H. M.D., "Atrial Fibrillation." The New England Journal of Medicine Volume 344:1067-178, No. 14: 5 Apr. 2001.

Fontaine, Kevin, MD, et.al. "Years of Life Lost Due to Obesity." Journal of the American Medical Association. 8 Jan 2003: Vol. 289, 187-193.

Haney, Daniel Q. "Hidden Factor in Heart Disease." *San Jose Mercury News.* August 4, 2002: A16.

Holmes, Michelle, D. MD, et. al., "Physical Activity and Survival After Breast Cancer." *JAMA.* Vol. 293, No. 20, May 25, 2479-2486.

"How I Stay Fit." *San Jose Mercury News.* October 22, 2001: B1.

Kolata, Gina. "In profound shift, death rates drop for heart attack, stroke." *San Jose Mercury News* January 19, 2003: A1. From *NY Times* News Service.

KPIX San Francisco, Tanner, Lindsey. "Study: Obese Young Men Can Lose Decades of Life." Aired on January 14 2003 at 4 p.m..

Krieger, Lisa M., "Cardiac Strain." The San Jose Mercury News. 3 Sept. 2003. A1+

Lyons, Julie Sevrens. "Survival of the Fittest." *San Jose Mercury News.* March 14, 2002: A1+.

Mitchell, T.L., L. W. Gibbons, S. M., Devers, and C.P. Earnest, Effects of Cardiorespiratory Fitness on Healthcare Utilization. Copyright © 2004 by the American College of Sports Medicine; 2004, Dallas, TX, 2088-2092.

Rauscher, Megan. VascularWeb. Http://svs.vascularweb.org/ _CONTRIBUTION_PAGES/Medical_News_reuters/ Atrial_Fibrilation_Conf...21 June 2005. Am J. Cardiol 2004;94:889-894. Rosenfeld, Isadore, MD. "Why Cardiac Patients Can Take Heart. *Parade Magazine.* Feb 9, 2003: 8–10.

Rosenfeld, Isadore, M>D> "Why Cardiac Patients Can Take Heart." Parade Magazine, 9 Feb. 2003: 8-10

San Jose Mercury News January 8, 2003: A6. From Associated Press News Service.

Stein, R., "Exercise shown to increase survival from breast cancer." The Washington Post, 25 May 2005

Sternberg, Steve. "Most Heart Attacks Caused by Unhealthy Lifestyle." *USA Today.* August 20, 2003: *SBC Yahoo News*: http://www.Yahoo.com

Study Links Sleep Imbalance to Heart Attacks. Yahoo! News. Http://www.yahoo.com 27 Jan. 2003.

Tanasescu, Mihaela, MD. et al. "Exercise Type and Intensity in Relation to Coronary Heart Disease in Men." Journal of the American Medical Association 288 (October 2002): 1994-2000.

Tanner, Lindsey. "Study: Obese young men can lose decades of life" The Mercury News, 8 Jan. 2003, 6A.

Wright, John W., ed. New York Time Almanac, Health and Medicine, New York Time, NY 1999. 376.

Index

www.ingramcontent.com/pod-product-compliance
Lightning Source LLC
Chambersburg PA
CBHW051443280526
45785CB00003B/1413